Homeopathic Method

For information on Churchill Livingstone titles, or to place an order, call:

UK: Freephone 0500 566 242
Europe : + 44 131 535 1021
USA/Canada: + 1 201 319 9800
Australia/New Zealand: + 61 3 9699 5400

For Churchill Livingstone

Commissioning editor: Inta Ozols
Project manager: Valerie Burgess
Project development editor: Mairi McCubbin
Design direction: Judith Wright
Project controller: Pat Miller
Illustrator: David Gardner
Copy editor: Christine Wyard
Indexer: Tarrant Ranger Indexing Agency
Sales promotion executive: Hilary Brown

Homeopathic Method
Implications for clinical practice and medical science

Jeremy Swayne BA BM BCh MRCGP FFHom
Dean of the Faculty of Homoeopathy, Somerset, UK

Foreword by
Conrad M. Harris
Division of General Practice and Public Health Medicine,
School of Medicine, University of Leeds, UK

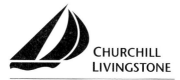
CHURCHILL
LIVINGSTONE

NEW YORK EDINBURGH LONDON MADRID MELBOURNE SAN FRANCISCO
TOKYO 1998

CHURCHILL LIVINGSTONE
Medical Division of Pearson Professional Limited

Distributed in the United States of America by Churchill Livingstone, 650
Avenue of the Americas, New York, N.Y. 10011, and by associated companies,
branches and representatives throughout the world.

© Pearson Professional Limited 1998

 is a registered trade mark of Pearson Professional Limited

First published 1998

ISBN 0 443 05926 8

British Library Cataloguing in Publication Data
A catalogue record for this book is available from the British Library.

Library of Congress Cataloging in Publication Data
A catalog record for this book is available from the Library of Congress.

Note
Medical knowledge is constantly changing. As new information becomes
available, changes in treatment, procedures, equipment and the use of drugs
become necessary. The author and the publishers have, as far as it is possible,
taken care to ensure that the information given in this text is accurate and up-
to-date. However, readers are strongly advised to confirm that the information,
especially with regard to drug usage, complies with latest legislation and
standards of practice.

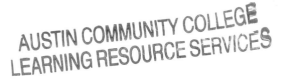
The
publisher's
policy is to use
paper manufactured
from sustainable forests

Produced by Longman Singapore Publishers (Pte) Ltd
Printed in Singapore

Contents

Foreword

It was brave of Jeremy Swayne to ask an allopath to write the foreword to his book. I neither give nor take homeopathic remedies; I am not happy when observation-based hypotheses are converted by inductive logic into 'laws'; and I find it difficult to suspend disbelief in the biological activity of ultramolecular dilutions. I am clearly in no position to assess the purely homeopathic aspects of the book.

It is not, however, primarily about homeopathic treatments, but about how homeopaths approach their therapeutic tasks. At this level, it has a great deal to teach conventional doctors, and I find it both fascinating and full of wisdom.

I came across the old term 'pathography' – describing what's wrong with a patient – in the writings of Oliver Sacks, and I saw that it was a neglected phase of research, tailor-made for general practitioners. Since then, trends in general practice have made it less likely that they will take up the challenge. It was a joy, therefore, to learn that pathography is not an optional extra for homeopathic practitioners, but an essential part of their methods, and safe in their hands. I hope they will make their findings known outside their own literature, as an important contribution to medicine.

It was a further joy that the book is so well-written – something uncommon in texts for doctors nowadays. The way in which complexities are teased apart, and fine and crucial distinctions drawn, is obviously the result of much reflection and hard thinking.

I recommend this book to everyone who treats patients. They will find it, as I did, an undiluted pleasure.

Preface

Homeopathy provokes a wide range of attitudes amongst its opponents and its adherents. Amongst the opponents two extremes are represented by the view, on the one hand, that it is a blasphemy against the god of contemporary science (Miller 1988) and on the other, amongst some fundamentalist Christians, that it is the work of the devil. Within homeopathy attitudes have been similarly divergent; they range from those who at times have viewed it as little different from ordinary pharmacology to those who see in it an expression of the divine life force. Most doctors who practise homeopathy in the UK are pragmatic in their approach to their work. They are simply impressed that it is a method that allows them to achieve better results for their patients than they could without it.

This pragmatism is nevertheless considerably enlivened by the excitement, perplexity and frequent astonishment at what seems to be going on. There is also no doubt that the clinical method, the homeopathic approach itself, enriches the professional lives of doctors who use it. This is partly because of the greater depth of perspective it opens up in our perceptions of illness and healing. All these experiences, the satisfaction, the excitement, the perplexity, have been part of my own use of homeopathy over the past 20 years. This book reflects them, and particularly the intellectual challenge of the subject; the questions it provokes and the opportunities it seems to offer for a better understanding of our task as doctors.

When presented with a book proposal, publishers want to know what audience the book is aimed at. This book is aimed at several audiences, but not just for the sake of a large market! My hope that it will interest different audiences lies in the reason for writing it. This is the desire to set out certain implications of the phenomena associated with homeopathy that to my mind do not receive sufficient attention, and that I believe to be of interest not only to students and practitioners of homeopathy but to all doctors and others interested in medicine.

Two phenomena

Broadly speaking we are concerned with two phenomena – the nature and effect of the homeopathic intervention and the biological process to which it is applied. Homeopathy is a tool that we use to engineer a change for the better in a patient's health and well-being. That is a very crude metaphor and will appal many homeopaths with its resonance of the mechanistic style of medicine that they so distrust. It is certainly a very subtle stimulus to call a tool, and its effects are far removed from what we usually call engineering. But the homeopathic medicine is a 'thing used in (our) occupation', to 'arrange, contrive, bring about', as the Concise Oxford Dictionary puts it, the recovery of the patient. I make the point in this way in order to distinguish emphatically the use of this tool from the other phenomenon: the biological process that is the dynamics of health, illness and healing.

The study of this phenomenon is not, of course, the prerogative of homeopathy. Samuel Hahnemann invented a tool that would influence these dynamics, apparently powerfully, and called it homeopathy. In developing and applying that tool over the intervening 200 years, homeopaths have been observing the dynamics of health in minute detail. The use of the tool has been for therapeutic purposes, but the by-product of its use has been to enrich our knowledge of the natural history of illness and healing.

Virtually all the attention within the world of medicine in general has been on the tool, the homeopathic medicine itself: on whether or not it is a real tool or a fancy focus for other non-specific therapeutic effects. Little attention if any is given to the phenomenon to which the tool is applied; to what is actually happening in the patient, and to the description of this phenomenon that homeopathy provides. The validity of these observations does not depend in the least on the nature of the tool.

Homeopaths, of course, are deeply interested in this phenomenon. This is for practical reasons, because their therapeutic method depends upon close attention to it, as well as for its own sake. But little has been done to describe the phenomenon and discuss its implications within the converse of medicine in general or in the context of the debate about homeopathy in particular. The conclusive demonstration of the biological activity of ultramolecular dilutions will be revolutionary. It is a thrilling or blasphemous proposition according to your point of view, and inevitably takes centre stage in the debate about homeopathy. But for the clinician, who is necessarily something of a natural historian, the phenomenon to be observed in the patient is in its own way as astonishing, and can be studied without waiting for that conclusive demonstration. This book attempts to do something to remedy this omission in the public profile of homeopathy.

A double agenda

Hence the book's double agenda and the breadth of its target audience. First it is written as a study book for students of homeopathy. Because other textbooks do not discuss the homeopathic approach in quite this way I hope it will help them to be aware of its wider implications, and to be able to explore these among themselves and with medical practitioners and scientists in general. They are a generation of homeopathic practitioners beginning their careers in an atmosphere of enquiry and acceptance that previous generations have not enjoyed. The book is written for experienced homeopaths too, so that they can debate and develop the ideas presented here. It is written for the general medical reader, closely or distantly interested in homeopathy, who may find the description of the clinical phenomenon intriguing and challenging. It is written for the sceptic in the hope that it will provide food for thought. And, although it does contain medical concepts and some jargon, I hope that these are scarce enough and transparent enough for the non-medical reader to enjoy and find some fascination in the account. Finally it is written for everyone who is interested in clinical method, in case taking, in clinical observation, in the consultation, in the doctor (clinician, practitioner)–patient relationship, in the story of people's illness. These are fundamentally important to the practice of homeopathy, as to all medical practice, and are a recurring theme throughout.

There are a few necessary points to be made for those using this as a study book. It is not about therapeutic method. It lays the foundation for it by discussing the information we need, and the observations we need to make to treat the patient. It deals with how to elicit them, the conceptual framework for them and the rationale for treatment that they provide. There are references to specific treatments, but these are only illustrative. So are the references to materia medica. Where specific medicines are mentioned in a particular context there are likely to be others equally relevant.

So the first agenda is to help those wishing to study and practise homeopathy. It describes the clinical method by which the prescription is chosen and its effect assessed. I hope that it will help practitioners to achieve good results through good clinical method. The second agenda is to draw attention to what more may be learned from the diligent application of clinical method to the study of illness and the healing process, which homeopathy exemplifies and which I believe to be one of the important contributions that homeopathy can make to medical science.

REFERENCES

Miller J 1988 In: After dark. Channel 4, 3 September
(Dr Miller spoke of his reaction to the claims made by homeopathy for the activity of medicines diluted beyond the point at which any molecule of the original material remains detectable in the solution as a 'profound sense of blasphemy . . . a blasphemous irreverence towards nature', emphasizing later that he used the word blasphemy in a heavily figurative sense. He described research that purported to substantiate the reality of this phenomenon as conflicting 'with the entire articulated structure of biophysics, of physical chemistry, and of our entire view about what the nature of molecular structures is'. Its conclusion, he suggests, 'requires you to disestablish the entire cantilevered structure of science'.)

FURTHER READING

Campbell A 1984 The two faces of homeopathy. Hale, London

Acknowledgements

Warm thanks to Erica Douglas, Michael Hart and Gareth Morgan for checking the text, to Alan Quilter for advice on style, and to my beloved typist and tea-lady, Clare.

Thank you, also, to Dr Eric Sommerman for permission to reproduce the case study on page 90 and to Dr David Reilly and Churchill Livingstone for permission to use the chart in Figure 10.1.

Clinical method in homeopathy and its general relevance in medicine

THE PHENOMENON OF ILLNESS AND THE HOMEOPATHIC APPROACH

The results of homeopathic treatment are often claimed to depend upon the practitioner's approach to the patient and the problem – the philosophical attitude, the style and content of the consultation, the time spent upon it. Few people deny that homeopathy 'works'. They agree that people get better. They recognize that changes occur that would not have been expected in the normal course of events – that is according to the expected natural history of the illness or the expected outcome of conventional treatment. For many, however, it is not the homeopathic *medicine* that works. The medicine itself is regarded by sceptics as a placebo, whose action is strongly enhanced by the context in which it is prescribed. If this is so, and it has yet to be conclusively proved that it is not so, we would still need to consider a number of issues whose importance has been largely overlooked because of preoccupation with the efficacy of the homeopathic agent.

The homeopathic method involves an exceptionally complete and detailed description of the patient, the illness and its evolution. It also involves a similarly detailed appraisal of the changes that follow the intervention. Thus it provides an unusually full account of the phenomenon of illness and the healing process.

Homeopathy describes a phenomenon that is real and significant, *irrespective* of the nature of the homeopathic agent. It is a phenomenon that we do not understand and that is very poorly described in any systematic manner in the contemporary literature of medicine. Homeopathy is a huge experiment in the phenomenology of illness and healing. We have hardly begun to explore and exploit its implications.

I believe that the correct choice of homeopathic prescription is essential to achieve the best results in homeopathic treatment. But I also know that the homeopathic approach is of great importance to the healing process and may often be responsible for the changes that take place. I am also fascinated by the phenomenon I am dealing with and the process I am involved in. If homeopathic medicines were to be proved to be placebos, that would not alter the fact of the therapeutic outcome, or of the value of the observations, which are an essential part of the clinical method.

The essence of clinical method is the process of enquiry and observation. Good homeopathy and all good medicine require that these skills should be developed to a fine art. This book is, in a sense, a celebration of that art, particularly but not exclusively as practised in homeopathy. And it is an encouragement to all practitioners whatever their discipline to make the 'small but significant shift in the way we see our work' (see below) that is crucial to our better understanding of it.

HOMEOPATHY, NATURAL HEALING AND PLACEBO

The extreme dilution of homeopathic medicines often extends well beyond the point at which any chemical trace of their source material will have disappeared. If they are indeed active agents in their own right the implications for our understanding of biophysics are challenging to say the least. By contrast the implications for our understanding of the therapeutic consequences of their action are not much different from those that follow from their presumed placebo action.

They cannot have properties that allow the same kind of biochemical control and manipulation of body function that is the pharmacological action of conventional drugs. For instance:

• The observed results of their action do not necessarily depend on regular repetition of the dose or the maintenance of a 'blood level' of the medicine (and there cannot be a blood level if there is no actual concentration in the medicine in the first place).

• Only the precisely chosen and correct medicine, or one very closely similar, will be active in the patient.

• Only a patient who is receptive to the medicine – who 'needs' it because of the similarity of the individual characteristics of their complaint to the characteristic prescribing indications of the medicine – will respond to it. Medicines will not act in patients who do not 'need' them – whose condition does not express the characteristics of the medicine. (But see discussion in Ch. 10, Getting worse.)

• The quantity of a medicine taken at any one time (one tablet or 50 tablets) is not significant. Overdose in this sense is not possible.

• Finally, the response in the patient is extraordinarily diffuse. It often involves conditions of mind and body incidental to the presenting complaint, and characteristics of the patient not directly related to the illness at all.

None of these things are true of conventional drugs. In their case the quantity administered and the blood level are critical. The only congruence between the characteristics of the drug and the state of the patient that is relevant to their action is their biochemical impact on their specific organ, system or pathological targets.

The response of the mind and body to the homeopathic medicine must be stimulated by it but does not use it nor depend upon its presence in the conventional sense. Indeed, there apparently is nothing present. It has no pharmacokinetics or pharmacodynamics, or none that are consistent with what we currently understand of the behaviour of drugs. This is perhaps homeopathy's only justification to be called a 'natural' medicine. The response involves the natural self-regulating functions in our minds and bodies, stimulated (mobilized, reinforced, integrated?) by the homeopathic medicine. In other words it is similar to the placebo response, the same as the placebo response perhaps, even if we succeed in demonstrating conclusively that it is not a placebo response, a conclusion that is getting steadily closer (Boissel et al 1996, Kleijnen, Knipschild & ter Riet 1991, Reilly et al 1994).

In either case, whether it is active or inactive, the homeopathic medicine is part of a therapeutic process that exhibits this phenomenon with extraordinary clarity – if properly observed. The essence of the clinical method of homeopathy is just such painstaking observation. This is matched by equally detailed study of the evolution of the illness prior to the homeopathic intervention.

CLINICAL METHOD

The phrase 'clinical method' is used here to describe the process by which we elicit the information we need to treat a patient effectively and to care for a patient well. The two aims are not identical, and it is worth distinguishing them because they make different demands of this process. It is all too easy to treat a patient effectively, especially with our present repertoire of medical interventions, but to care for them badly. Effective treatment does not guarantee good patient care.

'Clinical method' is also used as distinct from 'therapeutic method' – the therapeutic technique or agent used in treatment. To an extent this is a false distinction. What is described here as clinical method is in itself a therapeutic intervention. The process and the manner of the enquiry – history taking, examination, etc. – begin the therapeutic process and powerfully influence its progress and outcome. In some therapies, psychotherapy for example, enquiry and therapy are part and parcel of the same process. In osteopathy, hands on examination of the patient and manipulation may alternate without interruption. Many surgical procedures are investigative and/or remedial, depending on what is found in the process. Some investigations often have surprisingly therapeutic effects that are not an inherent part of either their purpose or the procedure.

In another sense every therapeutic intervention is a form of enquiry because it is an experiment whose outcome informs the continuing process of treatment and may enhance understanding of the problem and of the patient. The clinical process as a whole is a continuous cycle of seeking and responding to information, first in order to describe and understand the state of the patient (diagnosis), and secondly to take action that will change it for the better (treatment). But the two components of the process can be distinguished, and the purpose of this book is to discuss the clinical method by which the homeopathic 'diagnosis' and the indications and rationale on which treatment is based are arrived at.

In conventional medicine, diagnosis is focused on the nature of the illness or disease process. In homeopathy the concept is often applied to the task of identifying the appropriate homeopathic medicine as well. This is because the disciplines of enquiry, examination and (where necessary) investigation are similar, and because the characteristics of the drug, its materia medica or 'drug picture', are formalized and presented in terms very similar to the description of the clinical features of a disease or syndrome. Thus the diagnosis of the 'disease picture' and the 'drug picture' involve similar methods of enquiry and analysis.

We are concerned here with 'getting the picture', the process by which a complete and accurate description of the illness in the individual patient is built up, and upon which an accurate prescription can be based. It includes the evolution of the illness – the manner in which the patient's health has progressed to its present state. This may take into account the whole health history and its attendant biographical circumstances. Equally important is its continuing evolution, the changing picture after treatment, on which evaluation of the response to treatment and decisions about further treatment are based.

THE ATTRACTION OF THE HOMEOPATHIC METHOD

Many doctors who are introduced to homeopathy dismiss it out of hand because of its sheer implausibility. For some the implausibility lies in the proposition that medicines that contain no detectable trace of their source material can possibly have any biologically active properties. For others, it is in the individuality of the prescribing process, the diversity and subjective detail of the symptomatology required to identify the correct medicine for the individual patient. Then there may be the added implausibility of the alleged relationship between this detailed clinical 'picture' and the properties of the source material itself.

For many others, however, a steadily increasing number, this understandable scepticism does not prevail. Nor are they deterred by the limited evidence of the efficacy of homeopathic medicine from clinical trials. Many doctors, sceptics included, acknowledge that ignorance of the mode of action of a drug is no barrier to its acceptance. Many important drugs were introduced before their pharmacology was understood. Many doctors and most general practitioners (GPs) are more strongly influenced in their day to day work by clinical experience or by their local medical culture than by formal research evidence (Fineberg 1987, Greco & Eisenberg 1993, Greer 1988, Macnaughton 1995, Reilly & Taylor 1993). A number of factors may stimulate change in prescribing behaviour, for example, but it is clinical experience that determines whether the change becomes established practice (Armstrong, Reyburn & Jones 1996). It is clinical experience, at first or second hand, that persuades doctors, the great majority of whom in the UK are GPs, to take up homeopathy (Swayne 1987). GPs are more pragmatic and more eclectic in their approach to what makes sense and what works in medicine than their specialist colleagues. They are more inclined to base judgements on 'informed empiricism' (Pinsent R, personal communication, 1987), a kind of wisdom derived from experience refined by the intellectual disciplines of their medical training. They are more tolerant of what seems implausible (though even so, sometimes not tolerant enough), and prepared to put homeopathy to the test if it promises to pay clinical dividends. Those who persevere usually find that it does.

A powerful attraction for many doctors who become acquainted with homeopathy is its clinical method. Feedback from GPs who have followed training courses in homeopathy in Scotland reveals the extent to which the subject has revitalized their clinical practice (Reilly & Taylor 1993). The reasons why it is so attractive are important. First, it evokes and liberates vocational and clinical skills that too easily become dormant in contemporary medicine. It allows, indeed insists upon, an integrated view of the patient and their illness. Conventional medicine, separating us into different body systems each with their different specialisms and treatments, can make this so difficult if not at times downright impossible. Homeopathy requires that we take the patient's experience of their illness seriously in all its individual detail, in all its often implausible individual detail. For there is a great deal that patients want to tell doctors that seems too implausible or irrelevant to be useful to the medical model on which they base their actions. Homeopathy also offers the possibility of a response to aspects of the illness for which we would previously have little to offer. And all these things combine to produce a better relationship with the patient, which is the first prerequisite of good patient care on the one hand and job satisfaction on the other. These possibilities can be immediately attractive on first acquaintance with homeopathy; so much so that one doctor on an introductory course announced at the end of the first two sessions that it had been the most exciting day she had enjoyed for years. It is an excitement that continues to infuse the practice of medicine for those who continue to study and use homeopathy.

There may seem to be a degree of hyperbole in this last paragraph, so I want now to refer to another discussion of essentially the same theme from a different perspective.

THE IMPORTANCE OF NATURAL HISTORY

Conventional medicine has been very successful in identifying the common characteristics of specific disease processes. Epidemiology has helped us to understand the common elements in the causation of disease, clinical medicine the common symptoms, signs and syndrome patterns, and pathology the common manifestations in body tissues and structures. We are now also gaining knowledge of common cellular and molecular characteristics of disorder and their genetic foundations. These advances have been accompanied by progress in our ability to control and manipulate various stages in the disease process to our considerable advantage.

The precise detail of this process is nowadays chiefly conveyed in a profile produced in the laboratory or by some other technological analysis. The progress of treatment is similarly charted by the elimination or correction of these changes. The focus of attention is the pathogenic agent and the pathological process. Information that does not have direct relevance to these often has only marginal importance. Where a technical diagnosis of the presence or absence of physiological disorder is readily available there can be a temptation to bypass much of the clinical process altogether.

The consequence of this kind of analysis is that one pathway of discovery in medical science has almost petered out. This is the study of the natural history of illness, and of its corollary the healing process. We have lost interest in individual detail and individual difference, and in so doing have sacrificed the opportunity to achieve other new insights into the phenomenon of illness and healing that this might provide. It is worth considering whether the retreat from detailed clinical study of the natural history of our patients' state has deprived conventional medicine of an essential perspective of the whole phenomenon. Perhaps our ever-narrowing focus on pathological detail, down to the molecular level, has blinkered us to a more complete, and perhaps more effective, understanding of illness and disease. Is it possible that we are pursuing increasingly intriguing and sophisticated answers to the wrong questions? Be that as it may, it is certainly the case that the vital role of the natural historian is neglected in contemporary western medicine.

Detailed study of the natural history of the individual patient's problem is one of the most distinctive and important characteristics of homeopathy. It is essential to the correct choice and administration of the therapeutic regime, to the monitoring and interpretation of its effect, to any adjustment that may be required as the response proceeds, and to the assessment of its outcome. It embraces all the subjective and objective manifestations of the condition: its symptomatology and pathology, its clinical signs, its effect on function, relationships, mental state and creativity. It takes account of the whole equilibrium of the individual. The observations required of both patient and practitioner to yield this detailed description of what is going on are not intrinsically different from those required in conventional medicine. They are precisely the kind of skills and observations on which the early reputation of modern conventional medicine was founded, and which were critically important in the development of the art and science of diagnostic medicine 'until intellectual leadership in the profession was taken over by those whose work was based on a quantitative experimental approach' (see below), and it became increasingly possible to take diagnostic short cuts by virtue of easy investigation of underlying pathophysiological processes.

NATURAL HISTORY, PATHOGRAPHY AND RESEARCH

An eloquent plea for a return to the natural historian's role for conventional doctors was made some years ago in a lecture by Conrad Harris, Professor of General Practice at the University of Leeds. In the climate of modern technological medicine it was also quite a radical plea. He presented a number of the issues addressed here particularly clearly, and it is worth quoting generously from him (Harris 1989).

Early in the lecture he discussed reasons why the research challenge in general practice is not being met. One he suggested is:

the way that clinical work can become routine, leading to the loss of both curiosity and intellectual rigour . . . . It is easy to forget that every patient presents us, in a sense, with a research project in which we must gather data and reach conclusions. A good scientist goes to endless trouble to check for bias in his data and to check his conclusions, but clinicians do not work in this way. Sometimes they recognise patterns instantaneously; if not, they look for evidence that will support their diagnoses, rather than evidence that refutes them. The approach is defensible of course – in terms of clinical experience, a lack of time and resources and the patient's needs. We may also suspect that it is in the doctor's interests to stop asking questions once he finds a pattern he knows how to deal with, for going on may lead him into uncharted waters. Whatever the reason, we constantly throw away opportunities to learn something new.
. . .
Similar issues are raised in clinical management too, since every time we intervene in people's lives we are conducting experiments . . . . We develop routines . . . and come to believe in them, yet much of what we say is based on guesswork and ignorance. There is always a gap between what we know and what we need to know, and if we are not constantly exploring a little of it we are in danger of forgetting that it exists.

He warns us that: 'What we expect to find is powerfully conditioned by what we have learned . . . . This sets the limits of what we ask our patients about and the extent to which we are prepared to ignore anything they tell us that is not required by, or does not fit, a pattern with which we are familiar.'

Turning to the riches of potential research and insight to be found through natural history he says:

The observation and description of what is before one's eyes, unconditioned by preconceived ideas . . . are the starting point of all

scientific research . . . . When (observers and describers of living nature) are not valued it is a sign that their discipline is in the grip of dogma and that . . . whole fields will remain unexplored.
. . .
The natural historian has an honourable tradition in medicine, starting with Hippocrates and ending only when intellectual leadership in the profession was taken over by those whose work was based on a quantitative, experimental approach. The tradition can be revived, and we should expect medicine to benefit if it is.
. . .
There are no clinicians better placed than the doctors of first and continuing contact to observe and describe the common ills, and what is associated with their onset and their changes over time. The role of the natural historian is ours for the taking. It is but an extension of our daily work, fitting into its rhythms because it may be picked up and set down at will; it does not ask us to learn a new language or any special techniques; it needs only a pen and paper, a cross-referencing system *and a small but significant shift in the way we see our work* [my italics].
. . .
There is an old medical word . . . for the descriptive task I have in mind – pathography; and as pathographers, there is much for general practitioners to do. There is no shortage of work for pathographers, for in no condition has a final version of the natural history been written.

He goes on to quote some lines from Sir Thomas Browne, 'that urge a student to "join imagination, sense, reason, experiment and speculation in his studies . . . and so give life unto embryon truths and verities yet in their chaos." '

He even has a good word to say for anecdotes, recalling Frances Bacon's admonition: 'so knowledge, while it is in aphorisms and observations, it is in growth; but when it is once comprehended in exact methods, it may perchance be polished and illustrate and accommodated for use and practice; but it increaseth no more in bulk or substance.'

The whole lecture is a rich evocation of the excitement of the kind of scientific discovery that is open to all of us, particularly if we are willing to make that 'small but significant shift in the way we see our work.' It deserves to be read in full by medical practitioners of every kind. All doctors of first contact do have a special opportunity to observe and describe the common ills. But few, perhaps, find the time or more importantly the inclination to become natural historians. Those whose clinical method is informed by the precepts of homeopathy are particularly well placed to exercise this responsibility.

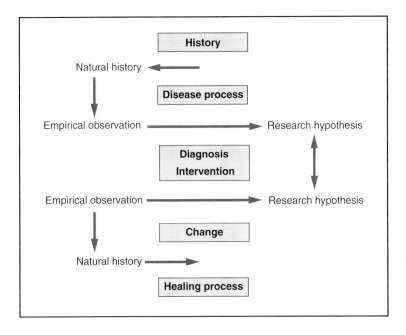

Figure 1.1 Pathography.

The role of pathography in the therapeutic process and in research is depicted in Figure 1.1.

THE HOLISTIC VALUE OF NATURAL HISTORY

The study of natural history is an essential perspective that homeopathy is preserving in contemporary medicine. It is important because it reminds us that illness is a phenomenon that cannot sensibly be reduced to its pathological elements, nor the art and science of medicine to the manipulation of these. It is important because it offers us the possibility of a better understanding of the phenomenon, and how we might better manage and respond to it. It is important, of course, for homeopathy because it is the source of the clinical indications on which the treatment is based.

It is particularly important because it gives us a way of perceiving patients in all the individuality, significance and meaning of their illness. This is the only view that can help us to do full justice to their medical need, that enhances the worship (worth-ship) that is an essential part of care. It is a view not only provided by careful attention to what is going on in the individual when they are ill, and all that has led up to it, but also reinforced by the study of the changes that take place across the whole spectrum of health and well-being as the patient recovers. This recovery will not always involve cure. It is sometimes more impressive when it does not. This is because of other subtle changes that enhance the quality of life, the whole equilibrium of the person, even in the face of persistent physical disability or disease, as when homeopathy is used in the treatment of congenital abnormality and in terminal care. Such observations give us a better perception of the meaning of healing, health and wholeness, and undoubtedly a better perspective within which to exercise our medical skills.

I do not mean to imply that clinical method is not painstakingly and perceptively applied elsewhere in contemporary medicine. It is of course alive and well and the mainstay of good medical education. But it is not always well applied. Sometimes it is skimped or devalued because of the exigencies of time (always the greatest enemy), the greater convenience of medical technology or the limited diagnostic or therapeutic perspective of the practitioner. When this happens opportunities are missed, the relevant skills and sensitivities atrophy, and perspectives are narrowed further. This problem was clearly stated not long ago in a leading article 'The importance of clinical skills' by J. Goodwin in the British Medical Journal (Goodwin 1995). The essence of Professor Goodwin's argument is expressed in two sentences: 'As far as treatment is concerned, it is the patient who must be treated, not merely the disease revealed by the result of the test', and later, 'Clinical skills and high technology must be shown to be inextricably linked'. He exhorted senior clinicians and those responsible for medical education, undergraduate and postgraduate, to emphasize these skills. And he warned that clinicians 'must not be complacent and should be worried that their skills are waning'. That small but significant shift in the way we see our work is an essential remedy to this state of affairs.

Nor do I mean to imply that the approach to clinical method that is concerned with individual detail and natural history is the be all and end all. An essential responsibility of the clinician, the first responsibility perhaps, is to identify destructive pathological processes that require corrective intervention, perhaps urgently. The finer points and richer opportunities of clinical method as described here may of necessity take second place in many clinical situations. But this kind of intervention must not become an automatic habit that neglects those finer points and opportunities. And indeed, inattention to clinical detail can of course cause us to miss the central diagnostic point, let alone any opportunity to understand the problem more fully.

E. F. Schumacher wrote about the distinction between science for manipulation and science for understanding (Schumacher 1995). Science for manipulation tends to degenerate into the search for power; science for understanding leads to wisdom. Medicine needs to pursue science for manipulation in order to exercise a necessary power over disease, but it must not do so at the expense of the science for understanding that true healing requires.

Professor Goodwin ended his article 'We must heed the desperate voice of the patient trapped in technology crying "Speak to me !" ' I would have preferred it if he had written 'Listen to me!'

THOMAS SYDENHAM

A fascinating historical perspective for the principles of homeopathy is provided by the work of the English physician Thomas Sydenham (1624–1689), credited as the originator of modern clinical medicine. His clinical method was based on minutely detailed observation of the patient. His reputation is said to have rested on 'his empiricism, on his refusal to accept any philosophy of medicine but rather his determination to observe and examine each individual patient with the open mind of a natural historian. Much of medicine's claim to a human approach and a concern for the patient as a person rests on the clinical tradition which Sydenham founded' (Marinker 1987). He taught us to 'listen intently and question the patient minutely about the march of events in the development of disease'. He regarded the manifestation of disease as 'an effort of nature, who strives with might and main to restore the health of the patient by the elimination of morbific matter'.

It is remarkable how much of Sydenham's teaching is reflected in the principles of homeopathy, though I do not know if any of its founders were consciously influenced by it. It is also serendipitous that Sydenham introduced Quinine (Cinchona) for the treatment of ague (malaria). It was Hahnemann's curiosity about Quinine, and his criticism of a monograph on it by Cullen that he was translating, that led to the experiment that was his first practical demonstration of the homeopathic principle. Repeated doses of Quinine induced in him the symptoms of the ague that it was used to treat.

THE NATURAL HISTORY OF HEALING

The concept of natural history is used in medicine to describe the natural course of a disease process when it is not changed by medical intervention. It is used here to include the natural course of the healing process following homeopathic or placebo interventions and in response to any non-specific therapeutic stimulus. The justification for this is the naturalness of the process whose history is being recorded, in contrast to the controlled behaviour of body mechanisms produced by most conventional drugs and procedures.

Summary

- The biological processes of illness and healing that homeopathy describes are independent of the nature of the homeopathic intervention.
- Homeopathy is concerned with self-regulation rather than pharmacological manipulation.
- Clinical method in homeopathy requires detailed study of the natural history of illness and of the healing process.
- This activity – pathography – is common to all medicine but central to the practice of homeopathy.
- Pathography is the starting point for all clinical research.
- The study of natural history is an essential perspective, which homeopathy is preserving in contemporary medicine.
- It is particularly important because it enhances our perception of the individuality and significance of each patient's condition and helps us to do full justice to their medical need.

REFERENCES

Armstrong D, Reyburn H, Jones R 1996 A study of general practitioners' reasons for changing their prescribing behaviour. British Medical Journal 312: 949–952

Boissel J, Ernst E, Fisher P, Fulgraff G, Garattini S, de Lange de Klerk E 1996 Overview of data from homeopathic medicine trials: report on the efficacy of homeopathic interventions over no treatment of placebo. In: Report of the Homeopathic Medicine Research Group. European Commission, Brussels

Fineberg H 1987 Clinical evaluation: how does it influence medical practice? Bulletin of Cancer 74: 333–346

Goodwin J 1995 The importance of clinical skills. British Medical Journal 310: 1281–1282

Greco P, Eisenberg J 1993 Changing physicians' practices. New England Journal of Medicine 329: 1271–1274

Greer A 1988 The state of the art versus the state of the science. International Journal of Technology Assessment in Healthcare 4: 5–26

Harris C M 1989 Seeing sunflowers. Journal of the Royal College of General Practitioners 39: 313–319

Kleijnen J, Knipschild P, ter Riet G 1991 Clinical trials of homeopathy. British Medical Journal 302: 316–323

Macnaughton J 1995 Anecdotes and empiricism. British Journal of General Practice 45(400): 571–572

Marinker M 1987 The chameleon, the Judas goat and the cuckoo. Journal of the Royal College of General Practitioners 28: 199–206

Reilly D, Taylor M 1993 Developing integrated medicine: the evidence profile, the postgraduate experiment. Complementary Therapies in Medicine 1(suppl 1): 11–12, 29–31

Reilly D, Taylor M, Beattie N et al 1994 Is evidence for homeopathy reproducible? Lancet 334: 1600–1606

Schumacher E 1995 A guide for the perplexed. Vintage, London, pp 64–66, 70, 118

Swayne J 1987 Homeopathic medicine in the UK: a contemporary profile. British Homeopathic Journal 76: 179–184

FURTHER READING

Bellavite P, Signorini A 1995 Is homeopathy effective (Ch 3), animal studies and laboratory research (Ch 4). In: Homeopathy: a frontier in medicine science. North Atlantic Books, Berkeley, California

The basic principles of homeopathy

These principles are only summarized here. Although some themes are developed more fully in later chapters this will be only in the context of the discussion of clinical method. The glossary supplies brief definitions of other important concepts. The Further Reading at the end of the chapter lists books that provide a more complete treatment of key subjects for those who are not already acquainted with them. This summary is simply intended to put the following chapters in perspective, and provide a framework for readers who do not wish to make a more thorough study of the principles described.

SIMILARITY

Homeopathic medicines act therapeutically in patients whose clinical picture is closely similar to the pathogenic effects of the source material of the medicine.

Homeopathic medicine is based on the empirical principle that substances capable of causing disorder, symptomatic, functional or pathological, physical or psychological, in healthy subjects can be used as medicines to remedy similar patterns of disorder experienced by people (and animals) when they are ill (Fig. 2.1).

This is the defining principle of homeopathy. It is not, as is often thought, the degree of dilution that makes medicines homeopathic, but the likeness (*homeo*) of the disease or suffering (*pathos*) of the patient to the pathogenic effects of the substance of the medicine. These include the acute or chronic effects of toxic

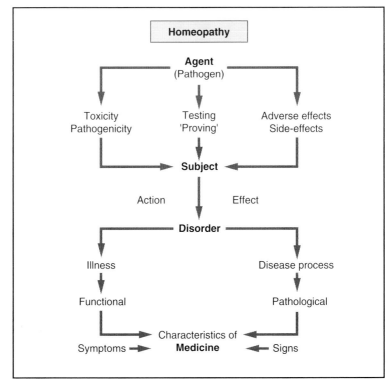

Figure 2.1   Derivation of homeopathic medicines from their source materials on the basis of their pathogenicity.

or pathogenic substances, and the side-effects of non-toxic substances in material (measurable) doses. They may be observed when the substance is taken accidentally or in the normal course of events (alcohol, for example). And they can be elicited when the substance is given experimentally in repeated doses to healthy volunteers, even in dilution. This process is called 'proving' or experimental pathogenesis. Substances that are usually benign or inert can also be tested in this way, and shown to produce an experimental pathogenesis. These observations are used to identify the potential therapeutic repertoire of the substances concerned (Fig. 2.2).

It is sometimes thought that homeopathy involves the principle of 'the hair of the dog that bit you' – the use of the *causative* agent as a remedy for the condition it caused. This is not

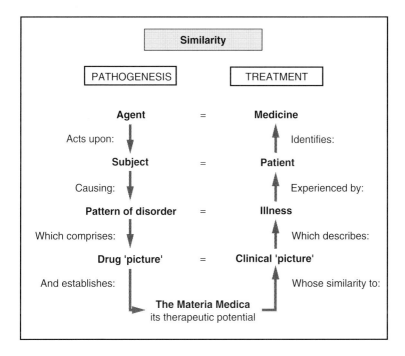

Figure 2.2   The relationship of similarity, which establishes the therapeutic potential of a pathogenic agent.

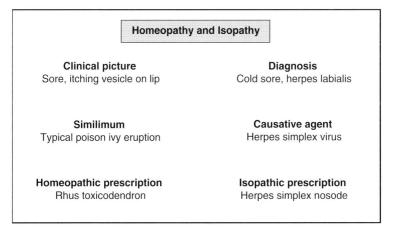

Figure 2.3   The homeopathic agent has effects similar to the complaint; the isopathic agent causes the complaint.

homeopathy (similarity), but isopathy (the same) (Fig. 2.3). Isopathy is, however, used therapeutically to good effect by homeopaths – preparations of grass pollen in the treatment of hay fever, for example.

Skilled homeopathic prescribing requires that the similarity of the characteristics of the chosen medicine should be as close as possible to the characteristics of the illness in the patient – the 'similimum'. It requires extensive knowledge of the materia medica and accurate pattern recognition to achieve this match. It is more akin to conventional differential diagnosis than to conventional prescribing.

VERSATILITY AND SPECIFICITY

Homeopathic medicines are versatile; a single medicine is useful in a number of body systems and a variety of morbidities.

Homeopathic medicines are specific to the precise form in which any type of morbidity is experienced by the patient.

The toxic, pathogenic and experimental effects of homeopathic agents are not usually exclusively organ, system or syndrome specific. The effects of any one substance may include multiple disorders of body and mind, and various permutations of pathological and functional states, gross and subtle changes, and concomitant physiological reactions. Again, progressive intoxication with alcohol is a familiar example, proceeding from subtle changes of mood, emotion and personality to grossly pathological damage.

Because of this diversity of pathogenic effects the therapeutic repertoire of a substance, its materia medica, will be similarly diverse – appropriate to a diversity of disorders in the patient that is similar to the range of its pathogenic effects. Thus, one medicine might be useful for treating depression, asthma, eczema or multiple sclerosis in particular patients if these disorders form part of its materia medica.

However, the characteristic effects of different substances on any one system will differ one from another. One substance will tend to produce burning pains, another sharp cutting pains; one will produce burning pain ameliorated by heat, another burning that is ameliorated by cold; one will produce moist eruptions, another dry eruptions, and so on. One medicine may therefore have great versatility in its therapeutic repertoire in terms of morbidity, but it will have great specificity for the behaviour of a particular disorder in a particular patient (Fig. 2.4). The repertoire of a medicine may include asthma but unless the effect of different weather conditions on the wheezing is the same in its materia medica as in the patient it will not be the correct medicine for that patient.

In conventional medicine drugs such as beta-blockers exhibit a kind of versatility comparable to this by virtue of their ability to influence a variety of symptoms and syndromes. They also exhibit some specificity in their application to particular presentations of angina or anxiety for example, though to a far lesser degree than would be necessary in homeopathy (Fig. 2.5).

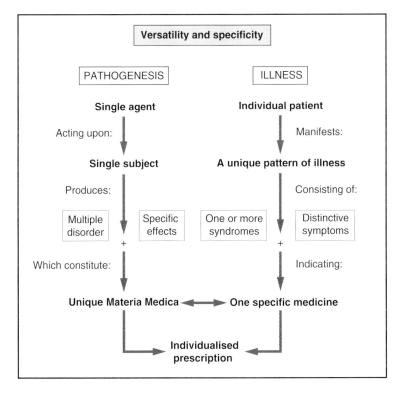

Figure 2.4 Homeopathic agents have a wide therapeutic repertoire defined by distinctive details of symptomatology.

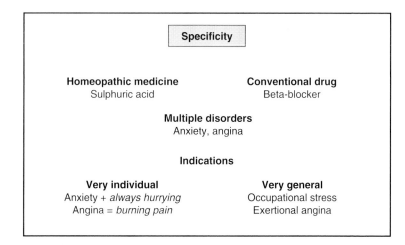

Figure 2.5   Homeopathic medicines are indicated by highly specific details of symptomatology.

And of course this versatility and specificity have no relationship to any pathogenetic action of beta-blockers themselves. They do not induce angina in healthy experimental subjects, for example. On the other hand they do induce unwanted effects in patients under treatment. This is their pathogenesis, but it bears no similarity to the condition it is used to treat. Iatrogenic illness is actually the 'pathogenesis' of the drug in a homeopathic sense. An excess of digoxin does cause a dysrhythmia similar to the fibrillation it may be used to treat, at least in terms of clinical characteristics. The homeopathic materia medica of *Digitalis* reflects this pathogenesis and this similarity.

INDIVIDUALITY

The correct homeopathic medicine must accurately reflect the experience of the illness in the individual patient and the individual characteristics of the patient him or herself.

This is a corollary of the specificity of homeopathic medicines described in the last section. The medicines are specific in respect of the precise details of the clinical picture revealed in their pathogenesis. Many medicines include asthma in their materia medica. Each one will reflect a subtly different clinical picture of asthma.

The same is true of patients. Many patients suffer from asthma but different asthmatic patients present distinctively different clinical pictures of asthma if studied in detail. Accurate homeopathic prescribing depends upon the correct match between the specific characteristics of the medicine and the individual characteristics of the illness in the patient. The prescription is thus said to be 'individualized' (Fig. 2.4).

The concept of individualization also extends to include characteristics of the patient's reaction to illness that are not pathological features of the illness itself. Thirst or thirstlessness, irritability or weepiness may not be part of the syndrome concerned, but they might be important defining characteristics of the state of the patient when it comes to selecting the specific homeopathic medicine.

Finally, it has been found both experimentally and clinically that patients with certain personal characteristics – body function, food tastes, weather reactions, temperament, etc. – respond with particular sensitivity to certain substances or their homeopathic derivatives. These 'constitutional' characteristics provide another facet of the materia medica and another route to the individualization of the prescription.

THE CLINICAL PICTURE

The concept of a picture is used in association with both the materia medica (therapeutic repertoire) of homeopathic medicines and the state of the patient.

The materia medica of a homeopathic medicine is sometimes called its drug 'picture'. The description of the patient's illness is called the symptom 'picture' or clinical 'picture'. This is because of the breadth of detail used to 'portray' the characteristics of the medicine and the ill person, which must be matched in choosing the right prescription. The word 'symptom' is used idiosyncratically in homeopathy to refer to any feature of the illness, even if it is an objective pathological state. Eliciting the clinical picture is like bringing together the pieces of a jigsaw puzzle, which must be then assembled into a recognizable pattern that accurately describes the patient. The complete set of pieces is described as 'the totality of the symptoms'.

To this totality may be added the wider description of the individual, their history and personal characteristics. In being encouraged to describe all this, the patient is often putting together a more complete picture of themselves as a whole than they have ever done before.

SYMPTOMATOLOGY

Symptoms are regarded as an expression of the dynamics of the illness, not just a pathological consequence of it.

Inflammation is one of the most fundamental healing mechanisms in the body. Its features are all expressions of the body's response to injury or insult – expressions of the dynamics of healing. They can be very distressing and we often seek to suppress them, sometimes mistakenly. Just as the symptoms of inflammation are expressions of a healing process, so the broad spectrum of 'symptoms' included in the clinical picture in homeopathy are seen as expressing the dynamics of the process by which the body or mind responds to disorder, rather than as the outcome of its failure to cope (Fig. 2.6).

The more dynamic the clinical condition the greater the scope of the healing reaction. Acute illnesses in an otherwise healthy person are often self-limiting because the system responds well in itself to pathogenic stimulus. Similarly, acute illnesses respond very quickly to homeopathy if we can make the correct prescription. Unfortunately our skills in acute prescribing are often poor because of lack of experience in their use in contemporary medicine. In chronic illness the dynamic state is weaker, more difficult to evoke and, with the progressive passage of time, often more difficult to 'depict'.

SENSITIVITY AND RECEPTIVITY

Receptivity describes the heightened state of reactivity possessed by the organism in its disordered state (when ill), its sensitized state.

Sensitivity is the ability of the organism to detect or recognize a particular stimulus.

The account of symptomatology and the dynamics of illness just given implies this sensitized state. The receptivity is expressed by the symptomatology. In the sensitized state the organism is

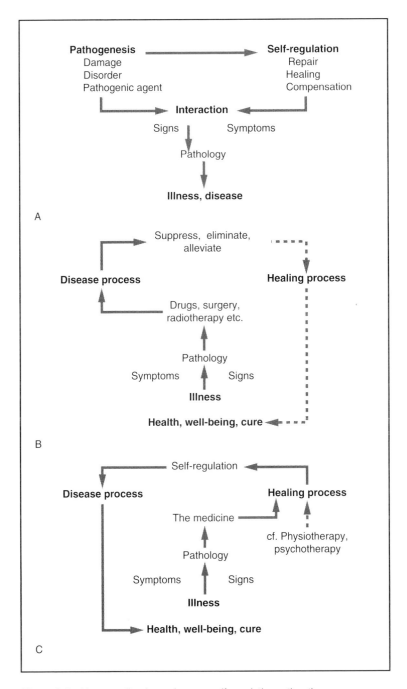

Figure 2.6   Homeopathy depends upon self-regulation rather than manipulation or control of the disease process.

responsive to the precisely corresponding homeopathic prescription, rather as a chemoreceptor is receptive to the precise chemical stimulus, though in this case there is no chemical structure involved.

During experimental pathogenesis (see Similarity, p. 17) and in treatment, some patients show more sensitivity to experimental substances or homeopathic medicines in general, or to certain substances or medicines in particular. Sensitivity to a particular substance or medicine has helped to identify certain constitutional types, those patients with a common set of personal characteristics who respond particularly well to a particular medicine – the Pulsatilla type, for example (see Individuality, p. 22). A general sensitivity can sometimes cause patients to react to incorrectly chosen medicines to which they have no receptivity, when there is no true correspondence between the medicine and the clinical picture. This is a rare example of a homeopathic 'side-effect'.

SUSCEPTIBILITY AND AETIOLOGY

Homeopathy treats the factors that predispose to illness as well as its manifestations.

Factors that determine the 'soil' in which the 'seed' of illness is sown, a correct perception of the state of the soil and its formative elements, are of great importance. These factors include the family history, past medical history, lifestyle, vulnerable traits (of personality, for example), life events and events that precipitated a change in the health of the individual. Prescriptions may be based directly upon these factors.

THERAPEUTIC RESPONSE

The response to treatment encompasses the whole of the patient. Change in the presenting complaint is not the sole arbiter. General well-being is an important consideration.

I once used homeopathy to treat a man with backache who not only became free of pain but immediately lost any further desire to smoke. The fact that he smoked had not featured in the consultation. This is a simple if crude example of the wide-ranging effects of homeopathic medicines. The fact that their role cannot be to manipulate or control because they do not have those pharmacological properties has already been mentioned; as has their apparent ability to stimulate self-regulation and self-healing.

Once mobilized this self-regulating process proceeds with its own momentum and in its own manner. The stimulus will affect any or every part of the system. Its field of action is the whole patient. The therapeutic response may therefore include any aspect of the patient's condition and constitution that is disordered or unbalanced. It will effect change in any order and at any pace, subject to certain principles which will be discussed later (Ch. 10).

The quality of the response is reflected in improvement in general well-being, in improvement of unbalanced states such as excessive appetite, extreme chilliness or a craving for specific foods, or in improvement in emotional equilibrium, as well as in improvement in specific symptoms. Thus assessment of the results of homeopathic treatment may include outcome measures quite different from a conventional assessment.

FURTHER READING

Boyd H 1989 Introduction to homeopathic medicine, 2nd edn. Beaconsfield, Beaconsfield
Coulter H 1972 Homeopathic medicine. American Foundation for Homeopathy, Washington
Koehler G 1986 The handbook of homeopathy: its principles and practice. Thorsons, Wellingborough

3

General issues of management

THE USE AND VALUE OF TIME

This is perhaps the most important and certainly one of the most expensive commodities in health care, and the most severely rationed. I once came across a quotation, which I cannot now trace, predicting that if effective treatments were developed that depended upon time the National Health Service (NHS) would collapse overnight. More than anything else it is what private patients are buying – time spent in consultation or time saved in waiting. It is one of the aspects of a consultation that patients most appreciate. Another is being listened to.

Listening is not, however, absolutely dependent on time. Patients can spend plenty of time with a doctor without being heard, and can know that they really have been heard even in a short space of time. What matters is the quality of attention that is given, whatever the time spent. The quality of attention determines the value of the time. Paying attention to the patient is therapeutic in itself. It is part of the 'worth-ship' mentioned in Chapter 1. But it has other more directly clinical virtues. It determines the quality of the information elicited. It encourages patients to give information because they feel that it matters and is respected. It makes it easier to discriminate between relevant and irrelevant information, to recognize when what seems superficially irrelevant actually is not, and to recognize what does and does not need to be pursued. If we attend properly to the patient we are more likely to realize whether more time is or is not needed, whether more time spent will be fruitful, and whether it needs to be provided there and then or can be postponed till later.

It is not easy to give our full attention. There are many distractions, from our own problems to the pressure of other people's, including a preoccupation with our professional technique and responsibilities. Paying attention does not require an intensely inquisitorial style of consultation, which may be inhibiting to the patient. The invitation in the practitioner's manner can be more effective than direct requests for information. Our attentiveness can give patients the impression that we have all the time in the world even when we have only a few minutes. Inattention implies that we really have no time for them, however long they spend with us. The difference may determine the outcome of the consultation and of our whole intervention.

It is a mistake to regard spending time with patients as a luxury, even when it is hard to find. If we do not give enough time and attention when it is required we build up a 'bow wave' of work ahead of us. This consists of unrecognized and unresolved problems that become more complicated, more entrenched, more diverse as time goes by, and hence more difficult to recognize or resolve. Enough time and attention given when needed can prevent this. It may be time spent listening, in physical examination, in teaching, explaining, or counselling. And time is often most needed and most fruitful when the problem is first presented. This may be when patients' motivation, courage and need, their anxiety, embarrassment and confusion are all most intense – when they are present in a complicated mixture from which understanding, hope and positive action need to be distilled. Or time may be needed simply to build the therapeutic relationship that will permit other work to be done at a later date.

The popularity and effectiveness of complementary therapies is often attributed to the length of the consultation, and sometimes rightly so, but it is not as simple as that. To be a good homeopathic prescriber it is necessary not merely to provide time, but to be a good clinician. It requires good clinical method based on attentiveness to the patient, making best use of the time available. It will be obvious from the chapters that follow that a great deal of time is sometimes essential simply to 'take the case': to elicit and record all the information in all the necessary detail to work out a correct prescribing strategy. This is particularly true, and perhaps not surprising in chronic illness. Homeopaths see a great deal of long-established chronic illness and always wish we could have seen the patient sooner. Eczema is one such condition. A report concerning eczema patients at a dermatology clinic gave an average duration of the condition of 17 years (Long & Finlay 1993).

Time is needed for other reasons as well. The acronym 'TEETH' has been coined for homeopathy by a sympathetic GP. It means, 'Tried Everything Else Try Homeopathy'. Because patients often do so as a last resort, generous amounts of time may be required to unravel the strands of past history and medical interventions. These may include many kinds of unresolved problem. A recent example was a patient with chronic minor illness in whom the devastating and still unresolved impact of the diagnosis and stillbirth of an abnormal baby 20 years ago was eventually revealed. It took 3 hours to arrive at this. Seeking homeopathy was incidental to her real need. This is an extreme example of a situation in which hours of time are required to resolve a long history of illness that would have been prevented by the proper use of time some years ago.

Many doctors are deeply frustrated at the lack of opportunity to give quality time to their patients. This should not be allowed to spill over into criticism of complementary practitioners who do. In fact, quantity of time is not always required in homeopathy if the quality of attention and clinical knowledge are good enough. Even spot 'diagnosis' of the right prescription is possible, and less complicated illnesses and acute illness may yield the necessary prescribing indications in a matter of minutes. It is easy, for example, to recognize an acutely feverish child requiring a prescription of Belladonna at a glance. I have given this to a furious toddler with earache on arrival at a night visit, and the child has fallen asleep before I had assembled my auroscope. A great advantage!

In some circumstances information can be acquired cumulatively. To some extent this always happens in any series of consultations in any discipline. No case history is likely to be complete after one consultation. But in general practice homeopathy, for instance, the clinical picture can be built up from separate routine consultations, often for different complaints. Just as any GP gets to know a patient and understand them better through a number of contacts over time, so can the GP homeopath accumulate the knowledge on which to base homeopathic prescriptions. This may not be as satisfactory as providing longer periods of time, particularly in recurring or chronic illness, but it is feasible, and can lead to very good results.

The time required for homeopathic consultations (or any kind of 'in depth' consultation) can be hard to find and expensive to provide. But if well used, and on whatever level the patient is helped, it should be a good investment for all concerned.

Box 3.1 is a summary of the key points relating to time and attention.

Box 3.1   Time and attention

- The value of time depends on quality rather than quantity.
- Time invested in a problem must be sufficient and appropriate.
- Insufficient investment of time creates a bow wave of problems that are incompletely understood and incompletely resolved.
- Quality of time is best achieved by giving the patient our whole attention.

ATTENTIVENESS

There are two kinds of attentiveness: a general attentiveness and attention to detail. The first is an awareness of the patient, which is the first step towards empathy. It is an open and accepting attitude that allows the patient to 'come across' as an individual. This is not always compatible with attention to detail. It may be necessary to sit back and focus less intently on precise observations; to allow the details to go out of focus so that the whole person is perceived more fully.

Attention to detail does, of course, require that intent focus on precise observations. This may involve systematic and painstaking enquiry and examination, but we must bear in mind the danger of limiting what we learn by the questions we ask or don't ask. It is important to encourage a free and spontaneous account of things from the patient, preferably at the beginning. The particular relevance of this employ in homeopathy will be discussed again later. The essential point to be made here is that our attention to detail must not be selective. We must hear and see, touch and smell if necessary, and often register emotionally as well, whatever the patient needs to communicate. We must not neglect the details that do not fit the familiar pattern, as Professor Harris says. We must not be fearful of those uncharted waters.

In the Organon, the treatise that first expounded the principles of homeopathy (Hahnemann & Dudgeon 1982), Hahnemann made two statements that are echoed in Harris's essay (see Ch. 1, p. 9). First he wrote, in paragraph 83, 'This individualising examination of a case . . . demands of the physician nothing but freedom from prejudice and sound senses, attention in observing and fidelity in tracing the picture of the disease'. Then later in paragraph 100, 'In investigating the totality of the symptoms . . . it is quite immaterial whether or not something similar has ever appeared in the world before', and 'the physician must anyway regard the pure picture of every prevailing disease as if it were something new and unknown, and investigate it thoroughly for itself, if he desire to practise medicine in a real and radical manner, never substituting conjecture for actual observation, never taking for granted that the case of disease before him is already wholly or partially known, . . . as a careful examination will show that every prevailing disease is in many respects a phenomenon of a unique character.' He is referring here not to disease in the sense of a specific pathological disorder, but to the illness experienced by the individual patient, to that patient's description of the totality of symptoms. Compare Professor Harris: 'The observation and description of what is before one's eyes, unconditioned by preconceived ideas . . . are the starting point of all scientific research'. And, 'in no condition has a final version of the natural history been written'. Unprejudiced attention to detail is the essence of good clinical method.

Both types of attentiveness described here are equally important to the quality of attention we need to pay to a patient. One or the other will take precedence at different times and in different situations. Different practitioners will employ them in different permutations. But we must be able to employ them both if we are to get the picture. This picture consists of the essential component parts, the relevant pieces of the jigsaw, but also the whole that is greater than the sum of the parts. The wider perspective is often necessary to a proper appreciation of the significance of each separate part. Attention to detail helps us to establish the uniqueness, and ultimately the worth-ship, of the whole.

This attentiveness is part of both the art and the science of medicine, which are themselves inseparable parts of the repertoire of clinical method. The interplay of art and science is expressed particularly well by George Orwell in his broadcast talk 'The meaning of a poem':

I have tried to analyse this poem as well as I can in a short period, but nothing I have said can explain, or explain away, the pleasure I take in it. That is finally inexplicable, and it is just because it is inexplicable that detailed criticism is worthwhile. Men of science can study the life processes of a flower, or they can split it up into its component elements, but any scientist will tell you that a flower does not become less wonderful, it becomes more wonderful, if you know all about it (Orwell 1970).

If we are to know all about our patients (or all that courtesy justifies and our responsibility requires) and realize how wonderful they are (despite all the exasperation, exhaustion and anguish they cause us!), we have to be truly attentive. In addition, giving our whole attention can have a remarkably catalytic effect on the progress of the consultation and the well-being of the patient.

Box 3.2 summarizes the key points relating to attentiveness and holism.

Box 3.2   Attentiveness and holism

- Paying proper attention is the basis of good clinical method.
- Attentiveness involves attention to detail and attention to the whole person.
- Paying proper attention establishes the uniqueness and worth-ship of the patient. It is therapeutic in itself.
- It is the attitude of the clinician, not the type of therapy, that justifies the label 'holistic'.
- An eclectic approach to illness allows the essential parts to emerge naturally from the whole.

AN ECLECTIC APPROACH TO ILLNESS

Some complementary therapists have tended to adopt the holistic label as their own, with the implication that conventional medicine is not holistic. This is unjustified. The willingness and ability to perceive a patient as a whole, to respect and respond to the whole that is greater than the sum of the parts, lies above all in the attitude of the practitioner to the patient rather than in the therapeutic method. A highly specialized technique applied to a circumscribed part of the body can be employed with complete respect for the person as a whole, and a full intention to make that technical contribution to restoring the greater integrity of the whole. A complementary therapy, even when based on a wide-ranging analysis of all the parts, can be applied without true sensitivity to that integrity.

But, if done well, the holistic style of the homeopathic approach has a particular advantage. This is its eclectic view of what is wrong. Having let the patient tell the tale in their own words, the process of enquiry ranges widely over the issues raised by the patient and also over many other facets of their life. It includes not only the health history, of course, and a review of any incidental symptoms and general body functions, but also tastes in food and recreation and reactions to weather and environment. It includes reactions to the circumstances of the patient's personal and social life as well, their relationships, emotions, mental state, intellectual activity, sexual life, and so on. Although these personal issues may not be presented early in the consultation they can be addressed at a later stage when the patient is more at ease. No greater stress is laid upon one particular facet more than another.

This broad and non-pre-emptive approach helps patients to see themselves more as a whole, and their symptoms or problems less as some separate and hostile entity. It also allows sensitive and difficult matters, often psychological, to be approached gently and within the balanced context of the whole. This obviates the uneasiness that can accompany discussion of what is and is not psychosomatic. It avoids that unhelpful duality of mind and body, and the temptation to take a one-sided organic or psychological view of the illness. At the same time it allows themes to emerge naturally and to establish their proper importance. If they then need to be pursued, that line of enquiry will have achieved its own natural momentum. Having had an interest in psychotherapy long before encountering homeopathy, I find this a very helpful way in to the exploration of psychological themes when the need arises. The broad spectrum approach of homeopathy allows the best possible view of the whole landscape and an effective means of identifying the most important landmarks.

THE CONSULTATION

Most of what has been said so far points to the fact that the consultation is the heart of the clinical process. This is so obviously true, and it is the focus of so much medical training. And yet the consultation remains a source of frustration to doctors and disappointment to patients. Lack of time, inattention and failure or lack of opportunity to respond to the wider 'picture' of the patient's illness, to the patient who is ill, account for most of this. Most of us in medicine are only too aware of the problem. But despite this we perpetuate it. Time is the chief scapegoat, and will continue to be unless we can demonstrate that, as I have suggested, time properly and more generously invested ultimately saves time. But I suspect we perpetuate the problem partly for another reason, which is that in fact we undervalue the therapeutic value of the consultation. The therapeutic potential of the consultation has been firmly on the general practice agenda since the pioneering work of the Balint groups in the 1960s (Balint 1964). This was exemplified by the book 'The doctor–patient relationship' (Browne & Freeling 1967), which powerfully influenced many GP trainees of my generation 30 years ago. Despite this the consultation is still too often regarded as just a means to an end; as the process that brings us to the point at which we begin to do something for the patient – the prescription, the investigation, the referral, the operation. We regard it as important, but as an important preliminary. Most doctors will insist that they do fully appreciate the therapeutic importance of the consultation. I am sure we do appreciate it. The question is whether we are able to exploit its therapeutic potential.

The consultation should begin or continuously reinforce the healing process. It will not repair the leaking heart valve or maintain the correct level of insulin. But it can ensure that the patient is best prepared for and most responsive to the specific intervention, and its repertoire of non-specific effects can provide an essential stimulus, or catalyst, to the mobilization of latent self-regulating and healing resources in the patient. This is the setting in which we prescribe the drug 'doctor', well recognized as a potent therapeutic (or possibly iatrogenic) agent, the central element in this repertoire of non-specific effects.

Until recently conventional medicine has been somewhat contemptuous of the therapeutic role of non-specific and placebo effects, though they are now being treated with increasing respect (Ernst & Herxheimer 1997, Oh 1994). For this reason we may have a tendency to play down their importance within the consultation, and hence the importance of the consultation as a therapeutic intervention in itself. Because homeopaths are constantly subject to the criticism that the consultation and not the medicine is the real therapeutic agent, they too have a tendency to play it down in order to justify the prescription. This is regrettable. All the research emphasis in homeopathy is directed towards proving that the *prescription* 'works' – that the medicine is an active therapeutic agent. This is certainly the most challenging aspect of homeopathy, because the most implausible. But there is a great deal to be learned from researching whether and how well the *consultation* 'works', and what effect differences in the style and content of consultations have on how well they 'work'. Homeopathy offers an excellent opportunity for investigating the non-specific effects of the consultation.

If I seem to labour the point it is because I believe it is important to establish the role of the consultation in the homeopathic approach as a legitimate and essential part of the treatment as well as the vehicle of the clinical method that leads to the prescription. As was pointed out in Chapter 1, clinical method is embedded within the whole therapeutic process, enabling it and contributing to it. It is essential that the consultation in homeopathy is seen in this light.

INTRODUCING HOMEOPATHY

In general practice we may be offering homeopathy for the first time to patients who know nothing about it. Patients attending outpatient clinics or private practitioners will often do so on their own initiative because of what they know or have heard of the subject. Whatever the extent of the patient's existing knowledge or ignorance, the basic principles should be introduced or reviewed, and if necessary discussed, at the first consultation or at appropriate times during the course of treatment. Many practitioners provide a written introduction of the kind shown in Boxes 3.3 and 3.4.

Box 3.3 Introducing homeopathy 1: what is homeopathy?

WHAT IS HOMEOPATHY?

The basis of homeopathy
Homeopathy is based on the observation that substances that are capable of causing disorders of the mind or body in healthy people can be used in dilute form as medicines to treat *similar* disorders in someone who is ill, whatever the cause of the illness.

This is the homeopathic *law of similars*, sometimes expressed as 'let like be cured by like'. The word 'homeopathy' is derived from Greek words for 'like' and 'suffering'.

The key to successful homeopathic treatment is identifying the similarity between the effects of the original substance in healthy people and the pattern of the illness in the *individual* who is ill. It is this similarity that is essential. The fact that the medicines are extremely, often infinitely, dilute preparations of the original substance is not the characteristic that makes them 'homeopathic'.

Choosing the individual prescription
The word 'individual' is emphasized because any particular disease or illness, although it may have a particular form of pathology, actually manifests itself differently in individual patients. The pattern of clinical symptoms and signs will differ in some details from person to person. This is true of the actual condition itself, but even more so if incidental factors like changes in mood, thirst, appetite, reaction to temperature, and other body functions are taken into account. The characteristic actions of the homeopathic medicine must match these individual characteristics of the illness if it is to have a therapeutic effect.

Although it does not always take a lot of time to identify these characteristics, it may require a longer and more detailed enquiry than you are used to, involving characteristics of the person who is ill as well as of the illness itself. It is not always possible to complete this at the first consultation, and follow-up consultations are important for building up a fuller 'picture' of the person and the problem, as well as looking for changes in the picture after treatment.

How does it work?
We do not know how homeopathy works. The fact that the medicines are usually so dilute that no chemical trace of the original substance could be present in them, makes any explanation on the basis of our present knowledge of physics or chemistry impossible. It is this fact that causes sceptics to argue that the benefits of homeopathy are due to the manner in which it is practised rather than to the biological action of the medicine – in other words, the 'placebo' effect. But experience has persuaded very many doctors around the world that this is not so, and formal proof that the medicines are themselves biologically active is slowly accumulating .

We know, however, that their action cannot be pharmacological. They cannot control or manipulate biological function in the way that conventional drugs can do. Their action is, evidently, to enable the natural self-regulating mechanisms in the mind and body to function more efficiently, and to mobilize and reinforce the healing resources, which already naturally exist. Choosing the right prescription is like choosing the precise key needed to switch on this process.

Box 3.4   Introducing homeopathy 2: the course of treatment

THE COURSE OF TREATMENT

What happens when treatment is successful?
The response varies from person to person and condition to condition. It may be rapid or slow. It may affect the main complaint straight away, or it may involve other symptoms, body functions or general well-being before the main complaint begins to change for the better.

Sometimes symptoms worsen before they improve, but such an 'aggravation' is not common experience. If it occurs it is usually mild, usually a sign of a good response and always settles down. It is very rarely bad enough to require any additional treatment.

We cannot control the response to treatment. The body is 'doing its own thing', and we have to trust it to know its own business. Nor can we focus exclusively on one aspect of a person's health and not another. We cannot choose to treat the patient's migraine but not their rheumatism, for example. We can only respond to the *whole* pattern by choosing the medicine that suits it best. The more accurate and complete the choice, the more complete is the response, and the greater the improvement in the general health of the patient.

Is it always safe?
Although it is a very rare event, an aggravation such as I have described can be severe. For example, a hay fever patient in one of the best formal trials of homeopathy had to withdraw because of a worsening of asthma. Such an event will require careful medical supervision.

Homeopathic medicines do not have 'side-effects' in the usual sense. Very rarely, unwanted symptoms that are not part of an 'aggravation' can occur, but are transient.

Patients who are taking conventional drugs should not stop these suddenly, or without the approval of both their general practitioner or other consultant and the homeopathic physician. Problems can arise from inappropriate changes of this kind. Collaboration between homeopath and conventional physician is always important, but particularly where conventional drugs are also being used.

Will you always need to keep up the homeopathic treatment?
This depends on the nature of the condition (how chronic, for example), and how well you respond. Often a condition will recover completely, and continued treatment will not be necessary, but occasional repeat prescriptions may be required if a condition shows signs of recurring after it has resolved. When a patient has several clinical problems, or has had problems for a long time, treatment may continue intermittently for years. In any case there are no long-term disadvantages in the use of homeopathic medicine.

THE NATURE OF HOMEOPATHY

At the first consultation I usually try to cover the following points:

1. We do not know how homeopathy works.
2. The medicines are too dilute to have the same sort of action as chemical drugs.

3. They evidently transmit some property of the source material, even though this is no longer present in detectable amounts.
4. This property stimulates the natural self-regulating mechanisms of mind and body to remedy the imbalance or disorder that the illness represents.
5. The choice of medicine is highly individual, based on matching the known characteristics of the medicine to the patient's own individual experience of the illness.
6. This requires a more detailed study of the illness and of the other characteristics of the person who is ill than in a conventional consultation.
7. The response to the treatment can involve wide-ranging changes in the person's health and well-being.
8. These are dictated by the body's own response to the medicine, which is not controlled by the prescriber.

These points take very little time to put across if expressed simply, and help to achieve a common understanding of what is going on.

The possible effect of this introduction on the patient's expectations of recovery cannot be ignored. It is one component of the therapeutic role of the consultation. We should not be sheepish about this provided we remain critical of the separate and different roles of the various elements of the whole therapeutic process. If the patient gets well we may not be too concerned about which element of the therapeutic process has achieved what part of the healing process. But only if we discriminate between the different effects of the various things we do can we learn to combine them more effectively for better outcomes, and better understand the phenomenon we are involved with. This is the creative tension between art and science in medicine, of which we need to be constantly aware.

THE SCOPE OF HOMEOPATHY: REASONABLE EXPECTATIONS

The introduction we offer to patients must include a proper awareness of what may reasonably be expected of homeopathic treatment. This will be a general review of the scope of homeopathy, rather than an assessment of specific changes to be expected from treatment in the individual patient. This can be made only when case taking is complete. Other doctors who are not acquainted with homeopathy as well as patients will also need this information. It is a good idea for homeopaths working in a consultant capacity, NHS or private, to provide this for GPs and specialists from whom they may receive referrals, or whose patients may refer themselves or ask to be referred. An appreciation of this kind can only be very general because expectations depend so much on individual factors. Whatever the pathology, the circumstances of the patient's life and the skill and experience of the practitioner will all affect the outcome. They will do so in any therapeutic context, but perhaps more so in homeopathy. This is because of the subtlety of its approach, the greater dependence on self-regulating mechanisms as opposed to medical 'manipulation', and the depth of knowledge required for the effective management of each individual patient even when they have common pathology.

An example of an overview of the scope of homeopathy for referring doctors is shown in Box 3.5. Ultimately a review like this needs to be based on research into comparative outcomes.

TIME-SCALE

Discussion of these expectations should include the time-scale of changes. In chronic illness the unpredictability of the time-scale has been mentioned already, but patients need to know for how long and how often treatment will be needed to achieve results.

There are three main phases of treatment, which can be described as the response phase, the recovery phase and the maintenance phase. The *response phase* involves the reaction to the prescription – changes in any facet of the patient's symptoms, general condition or psychological state that can be attributed only to the prescription. The pattern of change can vary greatly. It may or may not include improvement in the main clinical problem. It shows that something is happening and will indicate whether the response is favourable or not. The *recovery phase* involves change for the better in the clinical problem, which may progress slowly or rapidly. It may overlap or follow the response phase. The *maintenance phase* is reached when an acceptable outcome is achieved and remains stable with or without repeat medication.

Box 3.5   Selection of patients for homeopathic treatment

There is no condition that should be excluded from the repertoire of homeopathy, but certain conditions are unlikely to show the degree of improvement that can otherwise often be expected. These include major neurological conditions, cancers, endocrine disorders where replacement therapy is required and, of course, conditions where destructive organic change is already well established – including conditions associated with ageing. A long history of continuous or repeated conventional medication may also prejudice the response to homeopathy; as may personal, social or psychodynamic problems of an intractable nature. Nevertheless, homeopathy can have a palliative role in all these conditions, and will sometimes exceed expectations. It also has a role in supporting recovery from trauma and surgery.

For all these reasons, absolute 'exclusion criteria' for homeopathy are not appropriate when considering its general role and provision. Nevertheless, practicalities will often require a selective approach to the use of homeopathy, especially if it is to be effectively evaluated.

The following list gives a range of conditions well suited to homeopathy. Their suitability for treatment does not necessarily mean that they are easy to treat! The skill and experience of the clinician, and the dynamics of the illness in the individual patient, are important variables. Children often respond particularly well to homeopathy.

It is important to remember that in all cases homeopathy can be used in support of conventional treatment. They are not mutually exclusive. Of course, close collaboration is required to integrate the separate regimes effectively.

Disorders well suited to homeopathy
- Migraine and chronic/recurrent headache
- Irritable bowel; dyspepsia; peptic ulcer; some early ulcerative colitis; Crohn's disease
- Skin conditions
- Essential hypertension
- Dysfunctional gynaecological problems; PMS
- Glandular fever; post-glandular fever syndrome; chronic fatigue; postviral fatigue syndrome
- Asthma; allergic states and hay fever
- Chronic or recurrent URT/ENT conditions; incl. nasal polyp, glue ear, tonsillitis
- Early rheumatoid/osteoarthritis
- Anxiety; depression (not psychosis); some behaviour disorders (incl. learning difficulties)
- Chronic and recurrent urinary tract syndromes; prostatism; stress incontinence
- Recurrent susceptibility to illness; 'never well since' previous illness
- Intolerance of, or poor control with, conventional regimes

Each of these phases may have different pace and duration in different patients, and the quality of the outcome will differ in individual patients and different clinical conditions. In one patient with motor neurone disease the response phase was rapid, initiating a gradual recovery phase restricted to only some of the symptoms (movement of the tongue, ability to eat and swallow, salivation); the maintenance phase required continuous medication and was ended by the general deterioration in the patient's condition and his death. In the child with otitis media mentioned earlier, the response phase was immediate, the recovery phase a matter of hours and a few repeat doses of Belladonna, and the maintenance phase permanent without further medication.

The response phase may be no more than a few days in chronic illness but can be delayed for several weeks. The recovery phase may take years. The maintenance phase may involve full recovery with no need for further medication. Alternatively there may be partial recovery with intermittent recurrence of symptoms requiring occasional repeat medication or with some persistent symptoms requiring regular medication.

As might be expected, the longer the duration of the illness before treatment, or the more deep rooted a condition in the family history, the longer the recovery phase is likely to be. Prolonged treatment with regular or high doses of conventional medication prior to the introduction of homeopathy may also prolong the recovery phase and make treatment more difficult. For example, an average recovery phase of 2 years might be expected for severe long-standing eczema or asthma.

These are broad generalizations, but it is important to give patients some perspective for the time-scale of treatment. They need to have some perception of the difference between the direct mode of action of conventional drugs and the indirect mode of action of homeopathy, in which the time-scale is determined by the body's responses and not by the pharmacological properties of the drug. It may be appropriate to give some or all of this information at different times during a series of consultations, but the subject should be on the practitioner's 'Introducing homeopathy' checklist. Introductory notes dealing with questions about the course of treatment are shown in Box 3.4.

FOLLOW-UP AND CHANGE

With the exception of acute prescribing, effective follow-up of patients is impossible in homeopathy without good case notes.

Identifying and evaluating change in the patient depends upon comparison not only of the state of the presenting problem before and after treatment, but also of the concomitant and incidental features. The progress of the main complaint is often not the chief criterion of a good response. This may be inferred from change in other symptoms, general condition and body functions, and above all well-being.

Change for better, or worse, may be revealed and needs to be corroborated by review of many details that the patient may not recall having reported previously, or even having experienced. This will not be possible unless they are recorded. It is not uncommon for patients to report that nothing has changed, but for careful review of the notes to reveal that much has in fact changed, although the changes did not include the symptoms that most preoccupied the patient. Those presenting symptoms are not necessarily the ones of most importance to the practitioner. It is quite possible, indeed quite often the case, that a patient experiences an increase in the presenting symptoms but a marked improvement in well-being, which usually results in improved tolerance of the symptoms themselves. A patient with arthritis and prostatism and a minute area of psoriasis on one elbow returned after treatment with a fiery-looking scaly rash from scalp to feet. As I looked on in horror he said, 'Despite this I feel much better in myself'. His other problems improved quite rapidly, and he tolerated the eruption for 6 months as it receded gradually down his body, like the water running out of a bath. This was the most dramatic example of therapeutic aggravation and the so-called 'laws of cure' that I have ever witnessed (see Ch. 10).

Patients may also fail to recall the progress of symptoms *because* they have improved. This is often surprising because quite troublesome symptoms can be forgotten in this way. Unless the original state of the patient is described and recorded fully and well in the first instance the nature and significance of the changes that may occur cannot be elucidated.

The time-scale of change varies greatly and is unpredictable. It may be rapid, especially in acute conditions. But it may be very slow, either very gradual or delayed until some time after the prescription. It may not be appropriate to draw conclusions about the response to prescription for many weeks when treating chronic illness, and a month is a common follow-up interval. This requires patience from patients, and doctors, used to a short-term response to conventional medication.

Acute episodes will respond to the correct prescription rapidly. The speed of response can be expected to be in proportion to the acuteness of the condition. In other words, the response should be as rapid as the safe management of the condition requires. This will require equivalent care and frequency of follow-up. If the condition does not resolve progressively and completely a new clinical picture may emerge requiring a new prescription. If the response is not good enough or not rapid enough, the prescription will have to be reassessed and other management options considered. There is no reason why homeopathy should not be combined with other treatment methods in acute situations. Many GPs adopt a belt and braces approach. Because the response to the correct homeopathic prescription can be expected to be quick, a GP may give a conventional prescription, an antibiotic perhaps, to be dispensed after a specified interval if there has not been sufficient improvement. Close follow-up of acute episodes is important, both for the sake of careful management of the problem and in order to learn more from the response to the homeopathic prescription.

OUTCOME

A number of observations about the outcome of treatment have already been made – that it often exceeds expectations, that it involves aspects of the patient's health and well-being other than the presenting problem, that the time-scale and order of events vary greatly. All of these may need to be discussed at some stage. Patients often underestimate the therapeutic possibilities. It frequently happens that after patients have shown significant but limited improvement in the early stages of the treatment they are well satisfied with what has been achieved and do not look for further improvement. They are surprised, and usually delighted, when the practitioner intends to continue treatment, expecting to be able to achieve more. But this situation needs to be handled carefully so that practitioners neither impose their therapeutic optimism on the patient nor arouse hopes that are not likely to be fulfilled. Nevertheless it is not uncommon that patients' expectations fall short of the practitioners' actual and legitimate goals.

Similarly the possibility of change in other aspects of health may surprise patients, and the fact that the treatment strategy encompasses all their health problems requires careful explanation. There are difficulties for the patient involved in this, particularly if one of their problems is well controlled by conventional medication and another is not. Atopic patients frequently present for treatment of their eczema because it is poorly controlled and distressing, while their asthma is a negligible problem provided they tolerate the regular use of their inhalers. Homeopathy regards the effective treatment of both to be inseparable. In fact the recovery of the asthma takes priority over the eczema, being the more deep-seated condition by virtue of its involvement of more vital organs and its greater threat to health. Integrated treatment of multiple problems of this kind requires careful explanation, and sensitive negotiation to ensure that the plan is consistent with the patient's wishes and tolerance of change. It also requires skilful management and close liaison with the patient's other doctors or therapists. This is especially so when adjustment or reduction of conventional medication is involved.

These points emphasize the potential achievements of homeopathy and the need to deal appropriately with the implications of this. At the same time it is equally important to state that homeopathy is not a panacea. There is argument amongst homeopaths about how much it should ideally be expected to achieve if practised with the greatest skill, but generally speaking it is accepted that certain disorders do less well than others, and certain patients do less well than others. To some extent, as earlier comments have implied, these variations can be predicted, but we continue to find that some patients or conditions do better than we would have predicted, while others do not do well even though there is no apparent reason why this should be so.

NON-RESPONDERS: WHETHER TO PERSEVERE?

There are a number of possible reasons for the 'non-responder' state. One is always the possibility that we have not been clever enough, or attentive enough; that we have missed the point, the key indications that would yield the effective prescription. It is very difficult to know whether this is so. If we strongly believe that homeopathy should be able to help the patient we should logically recommend a second opinion. But one does not want to precipitate a patient upon another series of consultations if, in fact, the outcome will be no better. And yet when we do persevere ourselves we may find the elusive key that indicates a new and effective prescription. Two patients recently returned to me 10 years after presenting with their original problems, with important aspects of these unresolved but prompted to do so because of additional symptoms. In both cases a new prescription was found that transformed the clinical picture, leading to almost complete resolution on several levels – psychological traits, physical symptoms and well-being.

The clues to these prescriptions were available 10 years previously had I been able to relate them to my knowledge of materia medica, and had this knowledge been more complete. This kind of experience makes it difficult to judge when to give up. But it is important to do so, and to do so sensitively and tactfully when there is no prospect of improvement so that the patient is not committed to continued and fruitless consultation and can seek other help.

In passing it is worth pointing out that experiences of eventual success in treatment after a long period of disappointment and diminishing therapeutic optimism on both sides strengthen the inference that the therapeutic effect is not 'just' placebo. The non-specific effects of the consultation and the homeopathic approach, and the potential placebo effect of the tablets, have had plenty of opportunity to operate and have been undermined by continued lack of any response. The possible therapeutic effect of these factors still cannot be discounted, but it becomes harder and probably unreasonable to attribute the outcome to them rather than to the new choice of prescription.

(See also 'No change' and 'Intercurrent events', p. 177 in Ch. 10.)

QUALITY OF LIFE

Finally it is essential to consider the question of outcome in terms of quality of life. It is often necessary to warn patients with well-established and severe disorders, particularly cancer and neurological diseases, not to expect too much. Cure of the disease is very unlikely, but it may be possible to slow its advance, to alleviate the symptoms and to improve well-being. All this can be well worth the effort. The same applies to congenital disorders, including chromosome abnormalities, and hereditary diseases.

THE HEALING PROCESS

It will already be apparent that in describing the response to homeopathic treatment we are dealing with a process quite different to our common conventional perception of healing. But again it must be emphasized that the reality of the phenomenon is actually independent of the question of the activity of the homeopathic medicine. What is being observed is what is actually happening to patients, whether the active agent is the medicine or the enthusiasm of the practitioner, or any other combination of non-specific factors. Unless millions of people all over the world have been subject to a collective delusion for two hundred years, the phenomenon consistently described by patients and practitioners must be the healing activity of our minds and bodies.

Four characteristics of this process are worth summarizing here. The first is autonomy. Several therapeutic methods in conventional practice encourage autonomy in the healing process. These usually have the word 'therapy' in the title – psychotherapy, physiotherapy, occupational therapy, art therapy, for example. These aim to mobilize or reinforce the recuperative and self-healing powers of mind or body, or to encourage the stronger functions to compensate for the weaker. Chemotherapy and radiotherapy by contrast, and of necessity, act to control the behaviour of body cells, and most conventional medication and surgery acts to manipulate or control function. The response to homeopathy is closer to the action of the first set of therapies but exceeds them in the extent of the autonomy it demonstrates. The action of those therapies is generally directive, in that it proceeds by scheduled steps towards a predetermined and circumscribed goal. This is less true of psychological therapies, but true to the extent that they proceed by a set of psychological manoeuvres towards a psychological goal. These steps are to an extent managed by the therapist, however non-directive the approach.

The response to homeopathy cannot be managed in this way.

There are principles governing prescribing strategy that are intended to facilitate the healing process in different clinical circumstances, but how the body or mind proceed to act out the healing process is usually unpredictable and cannot be manipulated. The system is doing its own thing in its own way.

As has been pointed out, this process has its own momentum and pace of change. In acute conditions the response to a correct prescription is always rapid, but in chronic conditions any change may be rapid or gradual, immediate or delayed, progressive over a long period or relatively short lived. Changes occur in a sequence that has its own logic and will not necessarily conform to our wishes or priorities. Incidental symptoms or aspects of general well-being may well change before there is any improvement in the presenting problem. And some things may get temporarily worse before they get better or while others are getting better. Aspects of this sequence of change are described more fully in Chapter 10.

The second characteristic of the healing process seen in homeopathy is its multifaceted nature, once again shown most fully in chronic illness. There are homeopathic regimes such as the use of 'local' or 'pathological' prescriptions, which are targeted on a specific or localized lesion or disorder, but prescriptions based on the 'totality' referred to in Chapter 2, prescriptions based on the whole clinical picture, will have their effects on many facets of that picture. A recent patient presenting with migraine recovered not only from her headaches, but also from her irritable bowel and her long-standing nightmares. Even more locally focused prescriptions can sometimes have far-reaching effects, as in the example of the man with backache who stopped smoking.

The third characteristic is familiar throughout medicine and is known as 'syndrome shift'. This is the phenomenon in which one syndrome, usually a newly occurring acute illness, displaces a pre-existing condition, or at least its immediate manifestations. If the previous condition was chronic it will usually re-emerge when the intercurrent illness that displaced it subsides. The phenomenon is seen somewhat differently during homeopathic treatment when a more serious, deep-seated condition subsides while a less serious condition predominates. For example, asthma subsides while eczema increases, cardiovascular disorder improves while musculoskeletal disorder increases, depression resolves while physical symptoms increase. These are steps in the progress towards greater healthfulness of the system as a whole: examples of the so-called 'laws of cure'. The patient usually continues to progress, and the newly predominant syndrome subsides in its turn. Another example is the transient reappearance of the symptoms of previous, dormant disorders, or even, though rarely observed, symptoms of disorders that have been prevalent in the family history but have not hitherto been present in the patient.

The antithesis of this is a form of syndrome shift known to homeopaths as 'suppression'. Incorrect homeopathic treatment can itself produce this. A prescription focused too narrowly on an atopic patient's eczema may reawaken their dormant asthma, for example, even though the eczema is suppressed. This is a retrograde step, not proceeding towards 'cure'. The tendency of many conventional treatments is to suppress the condition. Homeopaths suspect that this results in the emergence of other conditions, possibly more serious, in their place. They recognize this form of syndrome shift in many patients, and make allowance, indeed accept the necessity, for some recurrence of the suppressed condition as the syndrome shifts back again, so to speak, as healing proceeds. This phenomenon needs to be confirmed and defined by research. My own most common experience of it is with a history of the onset of asthma directly following excision of nasal polyps, submucous resection, or clearance of sinuses.

The fourth characteristic concerns what we might call the 'personal dimension' of the healing process as opposed to the clinical improvement. The latter will usually lead to some improvement in personal well-being, social functioning, etc., but what is striking about the homeopathic response is that these improvements often precede clinical improvement. The patient that most vividly impressed this on me was a man in his late fifties with asthma of many years standing, requiring courses of steroids every few weeks. The most conspicuous benefits he reported from early treatment were the improvement in his relationship with his wife because of changes in his temperament, and the recovery of his pleasure in playing the violin. It was some time later that he became able to do without steroids, but in many respects he was already well.

Another patient with multiple sclerosis had previously been fond of bread and tea. When her illness developed she developed a marked aversion to these. The first change that followed homeopathic treatment was a recovery of her normal liking for these foods. There is no reference to these as familiar symptoms of MS though perhaps sufficient attention to detail in studying patients would reveal them. If so, we might gain some new insight into the nature of the disease. Be that as it may, this is an example of another level in the spectrum of change that extends from the frankly clinical to the intimately personal level described in the previous example.

Finally there is the extent to which the healing process we observe so often exceeds expectation. If the response to treatment involves the autonomous action of the body's own healing resources, this healing process must presumably be limited by the actual availability of those resources, the actual possibilities of recovery or renewal. Anatomical abnormality, destruction of tissue, deficiency of essential nutrients or metabolic components, for example, will not allow change for which these are essential, though a surprising degree of adaptation or compensation may be achieved. But, except in extreme circumstances, the possibilities of recovery often exceed our expectations or what the known natural history predicts. One of the lessons to be learned from homeopathy or from the working of the placebo response is that, given the right stimulus, the capacity of the body and mind to heal is greater than we commonly suppose. Because I am still partly conditioned by my conventional training and expectations, I am repeatedly astonished.

Box 3.6 summarizes the key points to remember when introducing homeopathy.

Box 3.6   Introducing homeopathy

- Patients and other practitioners need some concept of the scope and application of homeopathy.
- Homeopathic treatment involves perspectives and expectations that differ from the conventional.
- The different parameters and time-scales of change and outcome will need to be explained.
- Particular features of the healing process need to be emphasized: its autonomy, its multifaceted nature, transition from one pattern of symptomatology or syndrome level to another, and change in personal well-being.

HARD WORK

It is sometimes necessary to point out to the patient that homeopathy is hard work. It is certainly hard work for the practitioner who may spend literally hours of homework analysing a case and choosing a prescription. General practitioners who have taken up homeopathy often find it more intellectually and emotionally taxing, but less frustrating. One cause of strain is the uncertainty and sense of risk that can result from managing a therapeutic process that obeys the principles of autonomy described above and is not under the control of the doctor. It is hard work for patients, partly because they are much more actively involved in the therapeutic transaction, and partly because they have to adjust to the same phenomenon of autonomy in the healing process. They may have to tolerate therapeutic 'aggravations', and the syndrome shift already described. They may have to research their family history, which can be of great importance in developing a treatment strategy. They may have to recall and awaken painful experiences from their earlier life or significant life events that may have had a role in the aetiology of the current problem. Understanding these can be all important for choosing the prescription, as well as for resolving the psychological or interpersonal problems that may have persisted from that time.

The practitioner must keep in mind what is being offered to the patient and what is being asked of the patient. Both must be consistent with the patient's wishes, expectations and ability to cope. It would be wrong to imply that homeopathy always makes such demands of patients, but sometimes it does and some patients find it more demanding than others. This consideration is not peculiar to homeopathy, of course. Practitioners of any medical discipline must be sensitive to the impact and demands of the treatment as well as the illness upon the patient.

REFERENCES

Balint M 1964 The doctor, his patient, and the illness, 2nd edn. Pitman, London
Browne K, Freeling P 1967 The doctor–patient relationship. Churchill Livingstone, New York
Ernst E, Herxheimer A 1996 The power of placebo. British Medical Journal 313: 1569–1570

Harris C M 1989 Seeing sunflowers. Journal of the Royal College of General Practitioners 39: 313–319

Hahnemann S, Dudgeon R 1982 Organon of medicine, 5th and 6th edns. Jain, New Delhi, pp 73, 79

Long C, Finlay A 1993 Perceived underprescribing of topical therapy. British Journal of General Practice 43(372): 305

Oh V 1994 The placebo effect: can we use it better? British Medical Journal 309: 69–70

Orwell G 1970 The meaning of a poem. In: The collected essays, journalism and letters of George Orwell, vol 2. Penguin, Harmondsworth, pp 157–161

4

Case taking

SHIFTING OUR POINT OF VIEW

There is no fundamental difference between case taking in homeopathy and in medicine generally. The process of observation and enquiry and the kinds of information required are common to many other disciplines. The difference is in the range and detail of information. Specialist disciplines, because of their particular clinical focus, will be to a greater or lesser extent selective in their field of enquiry. There will be much common ground but an emphasis on particular parts of the landscape. General practitioners take the broader view, filling in different parts of the landscape on different occasions, cumulatively building up the fuller picture. Homeopathy takes a systematically wider view of most clinical problems, but the essential features of the landscape and the observations that require to be made do not differ in kind from those that will be addressed by other practitioners. What is required, and what makes homeopathic case taking different, is the 'small but significant shift in the way we see our work'.

Students of homeopathy can, indeed should, start to practise its skills before they consider making a prescription. They could do so without even knowing any materia medica. Similarly, any practitioner in any discipline can begin to apply its clinical method with no intention of practising homeopathy. The first step is simply to acquire the habit of adjusting our view of our work to reveal that little bit more of the landscape. The additional detail will permit either the formulation of a homeopathic prescription or the insights and discoveries, the research opportunities that Professor Harris refers to, or both. We must begin by listening, observing and questioning with this small shift in the focus and quality of our attention. Then we will register the hitherto unnoticed or previously ignored details, which reveal the individuality of each patient's problem.

This attitude makes impossible the 'collusion of anonymity' that Balint (1964) wrote about. It is a situation in which the person who is ill is lost as an individual because each doctor they consult sees only as much as he or she can conveniently cope with, the 'pattern he knows how to deal with', and never the person behind the pattern. There is an irony in the frequent use of the word 'case' in homeopathy because in other contexts it so often implies the antithesis of a person-based approach to clinical method. The practice of homeopathy begins by learning to perceive the individual characteristics of the illness and the characteristics of the individual who is ill. The following sections deal with aspects of this process. Once again it will be apparent that they are common to all good clinical method.

REFERRAL AND COMMUNICATION

The majority of patients seeking homeopathy in any consultant setting are probably still self-referred. Our NHS homeopathic outpatient clinics require referral letters, but the patient has usually initiated the process. This pattern is changing because an increasing number of GPs and even other consultants are recognizing that homeopathy has a legitimate place in the therapeutic repertoire they can offer their patients. Nevertheless the majority of patients are still likely to have taken the initiative themselves.

A referral letter is the first source of case material, but referral letters to homeopaths are often unhelpful. They may say so little as to imply that any information about the patient's history and health care is considered of no relevance to homeopathy – perhaps, even, none of their business! This is definitely not the case. But homeopaths are as much to blame as anyone else for this because they often do not themselves communicate effectively with the other doctors or practitioners involved with the patient. Good referral letters will be forthcoming only if the quality of their own communications deserves it. Homeopaths must demonstrate their clinical knowledge and competence, their perception of the patient's problem and the role of homeopathy in the overall care of the patient. Referral letters and reports back to other practitioners are all-important, not only for the clinical information they contain but also for the framework for collaborative care that they should provide. Having said this, it is necessary to add that the homeopath then needs to set this information aside for a while to allow a fresh and impartial view of the patient to emerge from their own story.

OBSERVATION

In all clinical situations, observation of the patient begins with their appearance and behaviour. This is essential to our perception and understanding of the person and the problem. It is the first step in the process, and can begin with the patient's first contact with the surgery or clinic (it has been well said that the consultation starts with the receptionist) and continue on their arrival in the waiting room or our arrival at their house. Non-verbal cues, manner of speech and use of language can be all important. In homeopathy these observations not only assist us in understanding the patient; they also provide possible indications for the prescription. They are pieces to be fitted into the jigsaw of the clinical picture. A neat caricature of this is the distinction between the crying of the child who needs Pulsatilla (who makes you want to cuddle them) or Chamomilla (who makes you want to smack them).

Boxes 4.1 and 4.2 show examples of the kind of observations that may be made and homeopathic medicines that might be suggested by some of these.

General observations such as colouring and texture of skin and hair, body odour, body temperature and sweatiness may be important in many clinical contexts, but are always relevant in homeopathy. The patient who takes off outer garments in a frankly chilly room because they are too warm, or who moves the chair away from the virtually imperceptible draft, may be providing a vital 'eliminating symptom' for the eventual prescription. Similarly, a sour body odour, greasy skin and hair, a tentative, cold and clammy handshake, easy blushing or flushing

---

Box 4.1 General observations of behaviour

Observing the patient
- Early, punctual, late? Friendly or unfriendly?
- Shy or assertive? Decisive or indecisive ? Talkative or laconic?
- Tidy or untidy? Relaxed or restless? Open or reserved?
- Posture, Gesture, Attitude

Indicated medicines
- Early   = Lycopodium   Late   = Calcarea carbonica
- Assertive   = Nux vomica   Shy   = Silica
- Tidy   = Arsenicum   Untidy = Sulphur

Box 4.2 General physical observations

Observation	Indication
Sour body odour	Magnesia carbonica
Greasy skin/hair	Natrum muriaticum
Dry, brittle hair	Kali carbonica
Sweaty handshake	Silica
Dry skin	Arsenicum
Moles, excrescences	Thuja
Long eyelashes	Tuberculinum
Flushed face	Ferrum
Easily overheated	Iodum
Sensitive to drafts	Kali carbonica

---

of the face, are clues to the 'differential diagnosis' both of the disorder and of the prescription.

SPONTANEITY

Not all patients can put their thoughts together easily or find the words to express them when first presenting their problem and may require prompting or questioning from the outset. This in itself may be a characteristic we need to take note of and to understand properly. Why do they find it difficult? Is it shyness, embarrassment, difficulty in recalling events, or difficulty in expressing themselves? Whenever possible, however, patients should be encouraged to talk freely and spontaneously about themselves and their problem; and without simply repeating what other practitioners have told them in the past. (Patients may need to be asked not to try to be too medical when telling their story.) The most vivid and individual features of the illness are often revealed in this way and the value of this will be discussed again later. Even when we ask questions we should allow the response to be as spontaneous as possible, framing the question in such a way as to encourage free expression of the answer, rather than constraining the patients to answering 'yes' and 'no' or to making a choice from answers that we have offered.

LANGUAGE AND MEANING

The language in which patients describe their experience is of the greatest importance. We must be prepared to accept and explore both its literal truth and its hidden meaning. If a patient says 'I feel like a lost soul', it would be a great mistake to assume that this is just a histrionic figure of speech. It may reveal a real need for spiritual help. If a patient describes a sensation of water trickling down his back, it is insufficient to write 'paraesthesia'. Similarly it is wrong to dismiss the description of the distribution of a pain or sensation because it does not conform to our knowledge of neuroanatomy. Sensations 'as if' ('as if water is trickling down my back') and symptoms that defy the logic of physiology and anatomy are often described. These descriptions recur in different patients time after time, and are found in the materia medica of particular medicines, and resolve with treatment. Their nature and significance may be elusive, but they cannot be denied.

On the other hand, vague statements may need to be elucidated more precisely. The statement 'I'm frightened of crowds' may represent simply a nebulous fear of all large gatherings. This can be a useful homeopathic symptom, but if there is more to it and it is taken at face value the essential point may be missed. The enquiry 'What is it about crowds that frightens you?' might attract answers such as 'I feel conspicuous in a crowd' or 'There are always thieves in a big crowd', which reveal much more specific anxieties with more precise indications. The question 'When did you start to feel frightened of crowds?' might be answered 'After seeing film of the Hillsborough disaster on television', with the particular fear and horror or the impressionable nature of the patient which that implies.

When the meaning of a statement is not clear it is helpful to restate our understanding of it in other words. This allows the patient to correct us if we are wrong, and may help to clarify the patient's own understanding of what they are trying to say. We must be careful not to put ideas in someone's head or words into their mouth but, when used perceptively and with care, paraphrase is a valuable aid to understanding and clarity of meaning. It is just as useful in clarifying specific clinical symptoms as more personal observations.

A common example of confusion of meaning is the answer to questions about the foods people like and eat. Practically everybody is now influenced by some belief, advice or anxiety about foods that are good or bad for us. As a result our natural tastes are subordinate to our 'better judgement'. But our natural tastes are as important as our attitudes, probably more so as they are likely to be more individual. Similarly, people may confuse foods that upset them with foods they don't like. They may very well thoroughly enjoy or even crave a food that upsets them, and consequently because of their habit of avoiding it say they don't like it. Such questions must be carefully phrased and the answers carefully explored if they are not to be misleading.

A particular example of the problem of language and meaning is worth mentioning. The concept 'delusion' is used in a broader sense in homeopathy than in psychiatry. In fact it is used in four senses. First in the formal psychiatric sense, usually associated with psychotic illness, with a belief that is inconsistent with the patient's actual circumstances or social and cultural milieu. Secondly it is used to mean 'illusion', which is technically a misinterpretation of an actual sensory phenomenon. And thirdly it may mean hallucination. (These uses need to be sorted out and clarified in the literature of homeopathy.) The fourth sense is the one in which it probably arises most commonly in everyday practice; this describes perceptions of oneself or one's circumstances that can arise as part of a neurotic reaction. For example, a person may feel without any justification that they have not done their duty properly, have failed in their obligations or responsibilities; or that they are ugly, too fat, or have very thin legs. Many symptoms described in the literature as delusions are questions of personal interpretation of this kind.

When a 'delusion' involves physical symptoms they need to be distinguished from sensations and objective observations. For example a person may *believe* without any evidence that their head is too large; or it may *feel* as if it is enlarged; or they or others may have *observed* correctly that it is larger than normal. This kind of distinction requires care in relating what the patient says and means to what the literature describes.

A final point about language and meaning is the general problem of relating patient language, doctor language and 'repertory' language. The problem of patient language and doctor language is familiar. Medical terminology and jargon easily confuse and alienate the patient. The language that patients use for referring to clinical matters may similarly confuse or mislead the doctor. A favourite example is the mother who was asked if her child was constipated. 'I don't know', she replied, 'He hasn't had his bowels open so I can't tell'. It is obviously essential that we ensure a common understanding of what we are saying to one another whatever the context of our work.

Repertories are books of cross-reference between symptoms and the homeopathic medicines known to be associated with them. They are used for decision support in choosing prescriptions. The problem of language inherent in them results from their origin in the relatively distant history of homeopathy. The language is sometimes archaic, and the changing historical context has affected some of the meanings and possibly the relevance. For instance, should the effect of 'riding in a carriage' on a patient's symptoms apply if the carriage is motorized rather than of the horse-drawn variety that was originally intended? An additional complication may arise from the fact that the early works were translated from German, the language of Samuel Hahnemann the founder of homeopathy, into English, which is now the common tongue of homeopathy. Contemporary revisions of the repertories are beginning to provide synonyms and cross-references between symptoms of similar or comparable meaning. This helps to select the 'rubric' most appropriate to the patient's experience, but much more work is needed to make the traditional literature relevant to contemporary experience. Meanwhile we need to explore the meaning of obscure and ambiguous symptom rubrics with experienced colleagues in the course of our studies.

ENQUIRY AND THE STRUCTURE OF CASE NOTES

Although the need to encourage patients to describe their problem and themselves as freely and spontaneously as possible is generally accepted, different practitioners employ different methods of enquiry. We all probably vary our method to suit the clinical circumstances and the personality of the patient. Both extremes of style of consultation are found. Some practitioners make a point of asking no direct questions at all, just prompting the patient to keep talking by free association. This method is used in the belief that the key features of the problem and the most highly individualizing characteristics will always be revealed this way. At the other extreme some practitioners use a formally structured method of enquiry to ensure that they do not overlook any aspect of the case. In between are various permutations of style and method suiting the personal attributes of the practitioner or adapted to the character of the particular consultation.

It is important not to be too rigid in our method of case taking. If we do we run the risk of pre-empting patients' individual expressions of their needs. Then we will never treat them correctly or care for them well. We must be responsive to the manner in which their stories unfold, using paraphrase and enquiry to enhance patients' presentations of them, and to complete them when they have no more to say themselves. We must be prepared to take diversions that lead us away from the point in question or the structured approach we may have in mind, returning to the previous theme at a later stage if necessary. A structured and printed format for case notes can still allow us to jump from topic to topic in this way, making notes under one heading or another as appropriate. Some practitioners find a formal record structure helpful. Others prefer a blank sheet of paper on which they write the heading for a particular topic as they come to it. Sometimes the results of this can appear fragmented and disorganized, with a note about a complicated aspect of a relationship following directly on from a note of the person's bowel action or dislike of strong winds. This requires coherent synthesis at a later stage, and care to review all the details and issues systematically during follow-up. The gain in insight from this approach can compensate for the occasionally chaotic appearance of the notes. Each of us must experiment, however, and find the method that best enables us to get the picture. The reference (p. 67) to the possible role of electronic patient records is also relevant here.

It may not be necessary to be as exhaustive in our enquiry as previous sections have implied. The clinical circumstances may not justify or permit it. It would clearly be ridiculous to explore the whole landscape of a patient's health and relevant circumstances in an acute clinical situation. That might be necessary later in order to avoid its recurrence or any continuing implications of the illness, but not at the time. On other occasions, even in chronic illness, we may be presented in a short space of time and within one circumscribed area of enquiry with such a vivid evocation of a distinctive clinical picture that we can confidently select the medicine it represents without any more extensive enquiry. These are further examples of the point made earlier that homeopathy does not necessarily require lengthy consultations.

Whatever the style or method we adopt for the consultation itself or the notes we record, we must nevertheless have at the back of our mind a conceptual framework for the picture we are trying to build up. As beginners it is probably essential to write down for ourselves the framework that best represents the discipline that we want to work to, however flexible the manner in which we implement it may be. Discipline is necessary to ensure the clarity of the information we have obtained, its accurate analysis and the eventual synthesis on which we will prescribe. As that discipline becomes second nature we may not need to keep it always in mind, but skilled practice requires it in the early stages and I find I still constantly need to remind myself of it.

EXAMINATION

Because so much emphasis is put upon the subjective experience of the illness, the true symptoms, there is a tendency in homeopathy to skimp or even neglect the physical examination of the patient. This is a mistake, first of all because as clinicians we must remain alert to all the implications of the patient's condition so that we may take all appropriate action. Even if a patient has seen other doctors, including specialists, in the course of the illness we should not assume that the problem has been fully and correctly construed and diagnosed already. Often it has, but that must not be taken for granted and if there is any possibility that some feature of the illness or some possible diagnosis has not been properly considered we should consider it, and undertake any further examination of the patient that may be necessary. On the other hand some patients consult homeopaths because they are shy or distrustful of conventional doctors for one reason or another. The patient may present a problem for the first time, never having consulted their own doctor about it. They will, of course, require full clinical assessment. One such patient presented with a mixture of chronic fatigue and anxiety, some history of bowel symptoms and a long-neglected recall for a cervical smear resulting from her reluctance to be examined. It took a long time to win her trust sufficiently to permit any kind of examination. When that was achieved she was found to have a fibroid the size of a rugby ball.

Homeopaths have excellent opportunities to pick up clues that may have escaped the notice, or may never have been brought to the notice of the regular medical practitioner. An example is a patient whose hypothyroid state was first suspected not in this case by a homeopath but by her acupuncture practitioner. This was a non-medically qualified practitioner and the story not only exemplifies the level of clinical acumen that any practitioner operating in a complementary role should aspire to, but also challenges the assumptions of those doctors who doubt the feasibility of non-medically qualified complementary practitioners exercising proper diagnostic responsibility.

This clinical responsibility is the first reason why the need to examine the patient should always be considered, but the observations will also be of value for the homeopathic case. Simple signs like the complexion, the state of the hair and nails, the length of the eyelashes, the distribution and character of body hair, the texture of the skin, the presence of moles and excrescences, the temperature of the body to touch, to name but a few, can be of importance as prescribing indications or as incidental observations to monitor during follow-up (Box 4.2). Many specifically 'clinical' signs will obviously not be revealed unless we look for them – the precise distribution and character of eruptions, the presence of heat in joints or swellings, crepitus, limitation of movement, rate and irregularity of the heart – the whole multitude of signs that form an essential part of the clinical picture. There is a great deal of pathology in the materia medica of homeopathic medicines, which the more modern tendency to emphasize the subjective and psychological features can tempt us to forget. The 'totality of the symptoms' includes the physical signs of pathological change, and we must look for these.

CASE NOTES AND CASE ANALYSIS

General impressions and detailed observations should be accurately recorded at or soon after the time they are made. It is a discipline we learn during our medical education, though in a formalized manner whose inquisitorial nature can be inhibiting if we are not careful. Thereafter our habits tend to become less diligent, and in general practice the record entries usually become minimalist.

Making notes can be a problem. The circumstances and pace of events in acute clinical situations may make detailed record keeping, even the recall of precise events, difficult if not impossible. In any consultation some impressions and insights cannot be expressed effectively in words in the notes, and have to be committed to memory. Writing notes takes time, and handwritten notes are often illegible, even to the person who wrote them. Nevertheless, good case notes are invaluable for several reasons. Without good notes we cannot confidently recapture the essence and detail of earlier consultations. We cannot review the march of events, or be alert to changes in detail that may be significant but overlooked if the original observation is not called to mind. (The word 'anamnesis', which is sometimes used for case taking, means 'calling to mind'.) We cannot review our judgements, decisions and actions if the indications and rationale are not highlighted. We cannot critically review our work and its outcome, use our experience systematically to learn more, or conduct research if the essential data are not recorded.

In homeopathy these reasons are all-important. The actual recording of detail is usually satisfactory. It is such a fundamental necessity for homeopathic practice, and the discipline is instilled throughout our training. But it is no safeguard against incorrect observations. The quality of even the most comprehensive notes is only a function of the quality of the observations that gave rise to them. Failure to record clearly and unequivocally the indications for the action taken, usually the prescription, is a common shortcoming. It needs to be remedied for the sake of our own work, but also to make it possible to share our experience and exchange help and criticism. Good notes are essential for case analysis, prescribing strategy, follow-up review and evaluation of outcome.

Case analysis is the skill that lies at the heart of homeopathic therapeutics. It has an intuitive element, as does all good clinical method, but this must be combined with and tested by intellectual discipline. It is an intellectual process similar to differential diagnosis, but leading to the prescription (Fig. 4.1). The skills and the information required are much the same – complete and accurate history and observations, clear appreciation of the significance and relative value of the information, the ability to recognize the familiar patterns and the anomalies, the ability to form hypotheses and test them, the ability to make clear decisions and to review them critically. Like differential diagnosis it is the step that prepares us to translate information into action.

Box 4.3 summarizes the key points of case taking.

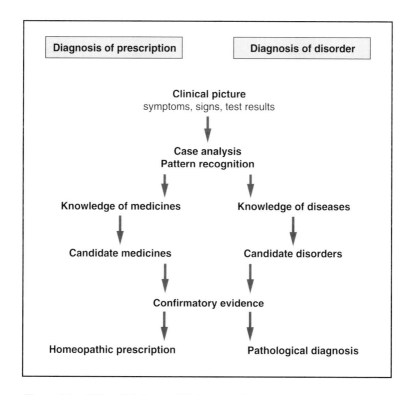

Figure 4.1 'Differential diagnosis' in homeopathy.

Box 4.3 Case taking
• The art of case taking in homeopathy requires a small shift in our point of view of the patient.
• Acute observation of the patient as a person is the first step in good clinical method.
• Care is needed to be sure we have understood all that the patient means by what they say.
• Case taking requires the right balance of structure and flexibility. Discipline is necessary but rigidity is inhibiting.
• The search for objective signs must not be neglected because of the emphasis on the patient's subjective experience.
• The complementary role does not absolve the practitioner of the need for good general clinical knowledge and acumen.
• Good case notes are essential for individual patient care, improving clinical performance, audit and research.

ELECTRONIC PATIENT RECORDS

A development that may influence all medical records for the better if it is introduced successfully is the electronic patient record. Computers have been used to record patient data in general practice for many years. Their use in hospitals has been less systematic but is becoming more so. The NHS Executive has adopted and developed the Read Codes as a standard medium for clinical information systems. These are a coded thesaurus of clinical terms designed to allow comprehensive recording of all information needed for the purpose of patient care, and from which data for audit, research and management can be derived.

As long ago as 1989 European homeopathic doctors involved in software development for clinical records and decision support considered adopting the Read Codes when they were suitably developed for implementation in homeopathic systems. Decision support systems to aid case analysis and prescribing have been well established in homeopathy for many years, though electronic patient records are only in the early stage of development. Ideally these developments should be capable of integration with systems for general medical care, as well as providing specialized functionality for specialist homeopathic practice.

Systems such as these, especially coded terminologies, will never be able to represent the full subtlety and narrative form of much patient information, but they will make reliable access to key information possible. The more subtle and informal information can be attached to the formal data as free text, and thus accessed indirectly via the formal data entry to which it relates. Systems using commonly agreed terminologies will permit retrieval, transmission and exchange of reliable and commonly understood information for patient care and any audit or analysis related to it. If their potential is fulfilled, they will have a major impact on case taking and case analysis throughout medicine. The development of homeopathy could certainly benefit from this. The use of computers requires clarity of thought and discipline in record keeping, which are desirable virtues in themselves.

These observations are something of a digression, and the possibilities will take some time to be realized. They are, though, relevant to the problem of clinical data collection in homeopathy. The need for this will become increasingly apparent in later chapters.

It may seem strange to place such emphasis on recording case notes after having written so much about the importance of paying attention to the patient. How is it possible to attend properly if our head is in our notes, or worse still we are occupied with a computer keyboard and monitor? This question has always concerned me because even in general practice I wrote copious notes, and have occasionally used a computer during consultations. But patients are not necessarily disconcerted by this. It depends on the quality of rapport that has been built up from the beginning of the encounter. If they are receiving good quality attention, if they are being listened to carefully and respectfully from the outset, the rapport that this creates does not suffer if the practitioner turns intermittently to the record. Continuity can be maintained while we do so. The art of remaining obviously attentive while writing is an essential consultation skill.

PERSPECTIVES

As we study a case, whether at the first consultation or progressively over a number of consultations, and as treatment unfolds, the patient's problems may be seen in a number of different perspectives. Separately or together these provide the basis for our treatment strategy. The aspects of the history that comprise these different views of the patient are explored in more detail in later chapters. This section presents an overview of the concepts involved.

Focus

Put rather simplistically, we may portray the patient in three depths of focus: close-up, wide angle or long distance. The close-up view focuses on the 'local' features of the immediate presenting problem – the skin eruption, the arthritic joints, the

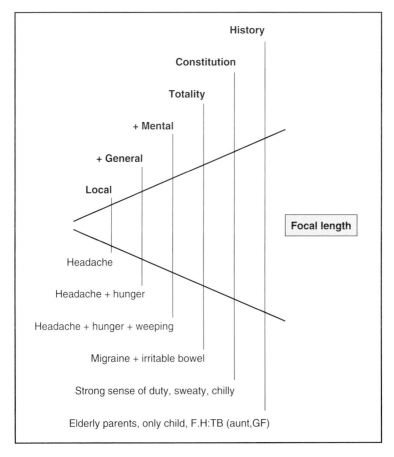

History

Constitution

Totality

+ Mental

+ General

Local

Focal length

Headache

Headache + hunger

Headache + hunger + weeping

Migraine + irritable bowel

Strong sense of duty, sweaty, chilly

Elderly parents, only child, F.H:TB (aunt,GF)

Figure 4.2   Different views of the history provide a differing focus for the homeopathic prescription.

headache. The wide-angle view progressively encompasses more of the patient – the general as well as the local features of the presenting complaint, the concomitant disorders, the constitutional features of the patient; the wider the angle, the more expansive is the view. The long-distance view includes the whole patient within the landscape and perspective of their lives. It encompasses their own and their family health history, and the evolution of the illness over time (Fig. 4.2).

The focus is reflected in the chosen prescription, which will have the same range and depth as the clinical picture. The close-up view will result in the choice of a specific prescription, a pathological prescription, an organotropic prescription or a local prescription. A 'specific' is a medicine reliably and consistently known to be effective for the precisely defined presenting disorder – the bruising, the insect bite, the panic attack. A pathological prescription relates specifically to the pathology – abscess formation, capillary damage, hepatocellular damage, damage to nerve fibres. An organotropic prescription, as its name implies, relates to a specific organ such as the liver, the spleen, the heart, the left base of the lung. Certain medicines also have tissue affinities such as synovium, periosteum or pleura (Box 4.4). The wide-angle view will give rise to a prescription based on the fuller clinical picture, the 'totality of the symptoms' or the patient's constitution. This may or may not be the same as the prescription indicated by the close-up view. The long-range view may suggest a prescription that reflects some influence in the past medical history or the family history. Again, this may be consistent with the clinical picture of the presenting problem and present health of the patient, but it may have specific reference to the aetiological factor concerned.

Levels

The 'focal length' analogy describes what we might call the horizontal axis of illness. It is a two-dimensional perspective determining how expansive, in terms of coexisting clinical features, or how extensive in time our view of the illness may be. Another perspective concerns the level or depth at which the illness afflicts the patient (Fig. 4.3). Previous chapters have mentioned the importance of the integrity and creativity of the personality as criteria of healing change. The syndrome shift

---

Box 4.4   Pathological, organ and tissue associations of homeopathic medicines

---

Pathological associations

Natrum carbonica	Sunstroke
Natrum sulphuricum	Concussion
Pyrogen	Sepsis
Calcarea sulphurica	Suppuration with discharge
Berberis	Renal calculus
Sabal serulata	Prostatism

Organ affinities

Chelidonium	Liver
Ceanothus	Spleen
Natrum sulphuricum	Brain, liver, left lower lobe lung
Crataegus	Heart
Hamamelis	Veins
Hypericum	Spinal cord

Tissue affinities

Hypericum	Tissues rich in sensory nerves
Calcarea phosphorica	Bone
Ruta	Periosteum, cartilage, tendons
Rhus toxicodendrom	Fibrous tissue
Arnica	Capillaries
Bryonia	Serous membranes
Nitric acid	Mucocutaneous junctions

---

between different levels of disorder has also been mentioned – in the interaction of different pathologies, as part of a therapeutic response, or in the form of suppression. These are examples of what we might call the vertical axis of illness. The horizontal axis plots the clinical and biographical events; the vertical axis plots the impact of these events on the health status and quality of life of the individual. The deeper the level of illness the more these are impaired, and vice versa. The pathology of syphilis, for example, well illustrates the evolution of a disease through progressively deeper levels, from the first superficial skin lesion to the eventual profound dissolution of mind and body.

There is usually a correlation between the 'vital' nature of the organ or system involved in the illness and the quality of life of the individual, but the most vital organ in this respect is the mind. Some might say the spirit. Many aspects of our being contribute to our unique individuality, including, as we have seen, our symptomatology. Our mind, personality and creativity define us most completely. This 'creativity' is nothing specifically to do with

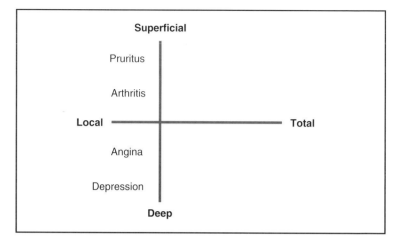

Figure 4.3 Levels.

artistic gifts, but includes whatever we bring to our role in life and our relationships that is life enhancing. In the conventional medical scheme of things the health of these attributes has not been a priority. Mental health care is notoriously undervalued and underresourced. In the homeopathic scheme of things this level of well-being is supremely important.

A patient might suffer from depression, asthma and headaches, and have a family history of tuberculosis. The headaches are a nuisance, the asthma restricts his physical activities, while the depression damages his relationships, his creativity and his whole enjoyment of life. Each represents a successively deeper level of disorder. The headaches might be the presenting symptom. The horizontal view would encompass these and might make them the focus of a local prescription. It would also extend to include the other problems and associated characteristics, enabling a prescription to be based on their totality. The longer view would recognize the three conditions as possible elements of the tubercular diathesis (a pattern of disorder associated with family traits and a particular aetiological factor, in this case the history of tuberculosis). This would prompt consideration of a prescription based specifically on the tubercular history.

The vertical view identifies the relative levels of the three disorders as a hierarchy of goals for treatment. Improvement in the depression should be the first priority or a necessary component of a satisfactory response if the patient is to be treated as a whole and the healing process is to proceed most effectively.

Layers

Some patients reveal a many-layered pattern of illness: different patterns of disorder superimposed one upon the other like layers of wallpaper. As one layer is peeled away in the course of treatment another becomes visible requiring a different prescription. The presenting pattern or syndrome gives way to another that expresses a further layer of disorder: a different expression of the fundamental imbalance or dysfunction in the patient. This does not mean fundamental in the sense that a disorder of biochemical function at the molecular level or a genetic abnormality is more fundamental than a cellular dysfunction or the dysfunction of a physiological system. It means a fundamental disturbance of integration of the organism or person as a whole. This cannot be reduced to or described in terms of particular and separate biological functions. In its more metaphysical mode homeopathy identifies this integrating and harmonizing principle as the 'vital force'. The next chapter will discuss the role of symptoms as an expression of the creative tension between integration and disintegration. Here we are concerned with new patterns of symptoms emerging as the healing process proceeds, expressing the next phase in the process of reintegration. It provides a new set of indications for a new homeopathic prescription to help the process on its way if the momentum of healing is not sufficient to carry it forward of its own accord.

Distinguishing 'levels' and 'layers'

The distinction between 'levels' and 'layers' is not always clearly made. The two terms are sometimes used interchangeably for the two concepts, but both have practical and strategic implications and need to be kept distinct. The example that follows (Box 4.5, Figs. 4.4 and 4.5) describes the two separate perspectives in the same patient.

Box 4.5 Case study: levels and layers

Mr N. L. was referred for treatment of irritable bowel syndrome. The most vivid features of the clinical picture, in fact the 'symptoms' with which he began to describe the problem, involved a long history of grief, emotional hurt and resentment. The history also included chronic upper respiratory symptoms, and the totality indicated the prescription of Natrum muriaticum (Nat. mur.). The choice was reinforced by the aetiology of the grief and by aspects of the patient's constitution. The focus thus included the close-up, wide-angle and long-distance views described earlier. The illness was reflected on different levels of disorder – the mood and emotions, the bowel function and the sinus congestion.

There was an excellent response to the first prescription. Well-being, mood and emotions improved greatly, sinus symptoms ceased and the majority, but not all, of the bowel symptoms resolved. This improvement was maintained over 3 months, but no further improvement was obtained with a repeat of the prescription.

At this stage dyspeptic symptoms began to dominate the clinical picture. They had occurred intermittently in recent years but were previously a relatively minor problem. They did not fit the Nat. mur. picture. Together with the unresolved bowel symptoms they did, however, correspond to a clinical picture of Nux vomica (Nux vom.). They also tended to be provoked by anxiety associated with competitive activities. And the competitive nature now appeared more strongly, although it could be glimpsed in the earlier history.

In conventional language he was now showing characteristics of a type A personality and the psychosomatic symptoms that might be associated with it. This, too, has features on different levels of mind and body, but represents a new layer of disorder, uncovered by the resolution of the previously dominant Nat. mur. layer. The clinical picture of this layer requires the prescription of Nux vom. The relationship of the layers is shown in Figures 4.4 and 4.5.

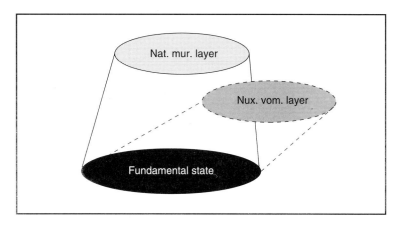

Figure 4.4 Different layers are aspects of the fundamental state of the patient.

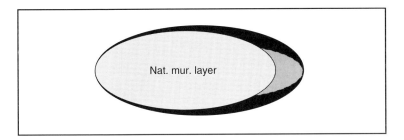

Figure 4.5 Dominant clinical picture superimposed on other layers at presentation.

Permutations of layers

The uncovering of another layer will not necessarily involve the emergence of a different disorder. It will often take the form of a new presentation of the existing disorder involving changes in the pattern and behaviour of symptoms. Some may diminish or resolve, while others become more prominent or change. The original disorder persists in pathological or diagnostic terms, though probably modified in severity, but with a new clinical picture. (Remember that a single syndrome or pathology can have many different clinical pictures.) This has been described already in terms of different pictures in separate patients, but it can arise in the same patient when another layer of the illness is uncovered. The different layers can be identified with the medicines that represent the different clinical pictures.

Many homeopaths regard acute illnesses not as circumscribed states but as manifestations of a chronic and more fundamental disorder even though this may be subclinical in the conventional sense (Fig. 4.4). Careful enquiry at a later stage would reveal the clinical picture of this deeper layer. This relationship between the acute and chronic layers of illness, whether the latter is overt or subclinical, is reflected in the acute to chronic relationship of pairs of homeopathic medicines. Thus Ignatia is recognized as the acute counterpart of Nat. mur., whose sphere of action is regarded as the more deep seated and chronic of the two. This pairing of medicines can be misleading as it implies that the acute medicine has a more superficial therapeutic role in general. This is not the case, and 'acute' medicines can act very deeply in chronic illness in their own right. But it does accurately reflect the relationship of the two medicines to separate layers of the illness in the same patient.

The coexistence of different layers may be recognized when certain details of a patient's case analysis do not conform to the prevailing pattern. That is to say they are not features of the materia medica of the medicine most similar to the pattern as a whole. They are pieces that do not appear to belong to the same jigsaw puzzle. It is possible that they may be hitherto unrecognized features of the drug picture of the indicated medicine. Just as 'in no condition has a final version of the natural history been written', so also in no homeopathic medicine has a final version of the materia medica been described. But they may be features of another layer 'showing through' the picture on the surface that predominates (Fig. 4.5). When this layer is peeled away (the layers of an onion is another metaphor used to describe this) these anomalous details will be found to be a part of the new picture that emerges.

The concept of layers can also be applied to a situation in which the essence of a problem is not being properly expressed on the clinical level. For example, a man may be unconscious of important psychological undercurrents in his life. (It is men far more than women who have the capacity for this kind of denial.) He presents with a physical disorder and even the most honest account of which he is capable and painstaking enquiry do not reveal any psychological unease. Following the first prescription, however, he experiences significant psychological disturbance for the first time. The source of this disturbance, perhaps in his earlier life, is eventually uncovered during follow-up consultations, and a different prescription appropriate to this far more profound layer of illness is required.

At first sight this example may seem to contradict the principle stated earlier that a therapeutic response and the healing process that results should lead from the deeper level of illness to the more superficial. Here it seems to have led the patient into deeper trouble. But in fact it has put him more in touch with himself. The layer that has been revealed concerns disorder at a fundamentally important level of his being. Unrecognized and unresolved it had power to damage him on other levels and inhibit his fuller development as a person. Uncovered in the course of treatment it becomes a source of healing for him.

The subject of layers of illness is complex and requires

continuing exploration at an advanced level of study. This discussion merely introduces the concept. It expresses a personal and by no means definitive view of the subject, which is one of many in homeopathy that deserves more systematic examination.

Evolution

The concept of the evolution of illness is not referred to in conventional medicine in so many words, but it is familiar nevertheless. There are syndromes and disorders that have different manifestations in different phases. Lupus erythematosus is one example. Here the early manifestations such as pleurisy, purpura or Raynaud's phenomenon may be associated with the underlying disease only retrospectively once it is more fully developed. The changing clinical picture in these disorders may be due to the progressively destructive nature of the disease or to its long-term complications. Syphilis is another example of a progressively destructive disease process. Rheumatic fever and diabetes are examples of processes whose evolution produces secondary complications. Another evolutionary pattern involves the common aetiological origin of a history of separate illnesses. Smoking is a notorious example of a single aetiological cause for a variety of different disorders (respiratory, gastrointestinal, cardiovascular) that could occur in one patient at different times.

These particular 'evolutionary' possibilities are well recognized in medicine, but unless a common thread of this kind is detected the separate illnesses that occur at different stages of our lives are seen as unrelated episodes. In homeopathy, on the other hand, the evolutionary perspective is always important.

All the chronologically separate episodes, whatever the different systems involved and however different the pathologies, are seen as elements in a single coherent pattern of disorder (Box 4.6). These separate elements need to be integrated in our interpretation of the patient's history and of the current clinical picture, just as we would form an integrated view of separate events in the evolution of a complex syndrome like lupus erythematosus from a conventional point of view. Such an evolutionary perspective makes sense of past events and present problems. It assists diagnosis and informs our treatment strategy. Conventionally unless there is an aetiological link, possibly psychosomatic, we would not form a similarly integrated view of a history of, for example, recurrent sore throat and adenitis in childhood, migraine in the late teens and rheumatoid arthritis in adult life. In homeopathy we would do so.

Box 4.6   Case study: evolution

Figure 4.6 depicts the medical history of a patient throughout her life. She presented in her 60s with a 15-year history of perianal soreness, unrelieved by conventional treatments. It shows the early atopic pattern, with eczema dying out and then recurring mildly in later life. Asthma developed after tonsillectomy and ceased at the age of 20 but was immediately followed by the onset of migraine. Escalating gynaecological problems developed throughout adult life until she had a hysterectomy. Hay fever succeeded the asthma and eczema. Vaginitis continued after hysterectomy, eventually seeming to give way to the perianal condition, probably related to her eczema.

The family history presents a number of predisposing factors. (The aetiological significance of such factors and their relevance to prescribing strategy are discussed elsewhere in this book.)

The pattern shows a changing dominance of different syndromes at different stages. The asthma resolved to be immediately succeeded by migraine, a less threatening condition. Following hysterectomy the whole pattern progressed to milder and more superficial manifestations of disorder, and the patient reported progressively improving well-being in middle age. In other words, the history showed a favourable 'direction of cure'.

This concept will be discussed more fully later. It describes a favourable sequence of change in the clinical picture in response to homeopathic treatment. In this patient's case, however, the interventions prior to the consultation for perianal soreness had all been conventional. There is a tendency amongst complementary practitioners to assume that most conventional medicine is not conducive to a positive 'direction of cure'. This case suggests that that assumption requires critical examination. The dynamics of illness and their evolution can be influenced by many kinds of circumstance and intervention. It is a matter of speculation as to what accounts for this patient's progressively improving health. Detailed pathography might provide some clues in this particular case. Detailed enquiry of that kind may enhance our understanding of disease processes in general.

Another condition of which we would conventionally take an integrated view is atopy. Despite the differences in pathology we recognize the coexistent or alternating eczema and asthma as facets of a single underlying trait, and we would expect to find the same trait in the family history. This is a good conventional example of a phenomenon that is thought to be pervasive in homeopathy: a trait that links different disorders in the present and the past, including previous generations.

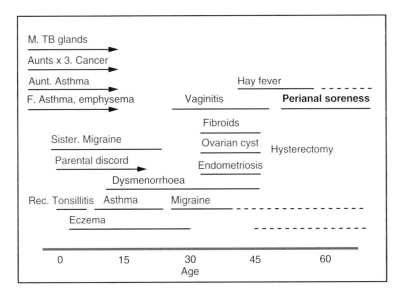

Figure 4.6 Evolution of a medical history.

So far this has been a static view of the relationship between different illnesses in our life history. Evolution is dynamic and we are interested not just in the occurrence of different disorders but the process of transition from one to another. We are concerned with types of disorder that occur in one patient at the same time or from time to time, and the association between them, and in the progress from one to another. Syndrome shift, changing levels and the emergence of multiple layers are all part of this.

The evolution of the illness can lead us to the prescription. This is because the pathogenesis of the medicine shows the same evolution and the 'law of similars' is in operation again. We may know this in two ways. The experimental or natural pathogenesis, or the toxicology of the agent from which the medicine is derived (see Ch. 2), may have shown the same progression and sequence of symptomatic and pathological change as we see in the patient. Or clinical experience with the medicine may have demonstrated its usefulness in situations where this same progression of clinical states is found.

In summary, the evolution of the case is the dynamic relationship between episodes of illness in the course of a patient's life and possibly family history, of which the current clinical picture is the culmination.

Traits and miasms

The previous sections have mentioned aetiological factors that influence our personal and family health history and traits that underlie that history and constitute the relationship between its separate events. In homeopathic jargon, these common evolutionary threads are often described as 'miasms'. In common use this means an 'infectious or noxious emanation' (Concise Oxford Dictionary), such as the mist arising from a malarial swamp. The Greek origin of the word means 'pollution', and it quite graphically suggests some pervasive influence that is the source of all the illness in an individual. A great deal can be and has been written about miasms. The concept and its various theories deserve to be studied because of the light they may shed on mechanisms of illness if systematically investigated. In the context of this book it is necessary only to be aware of its use in describing the patterns of illness and their development over time that are observed when studying our patients. Three main patterns are described – underactivity and instability (labelled Psora), overactivity (labelled Sycosis) and breakdown, collapse and degeneration (labelled Syphilis because of the original association with the manifestations of that disease). Certain homeopathic medicines are associated with one or more of these patterns.

CONCLUSION

This section has presented different perspectives that we may use to construe the illness. They are helpful in three ways: in interpreting the illness and its origins in this particular patient, in identifying a possible prescription, and in considering the prognosis – how much work needs to be done and what it may be possible to achieve.

Interestingly, and perhaps not surprisingly, an acceptable interpretation of the illness is what many patients consulting for homeopathy are seeking in addition to effective treatment. They will say that they want to know what is really wrong with them and why they are ill. They have realized that conventional diagnosis provides a description of the pathological nature of their illness, where this can be defined, but often explains little if anything of its origins, why they have become ill in this way at this time, or why the illness is taking this particular course. Where no pathological explanation for their illness is available, or active pathology has been excluded, far from being reassured they may remain anxious, certainly perplexed and, of course, still feeling ill.

We should not pretend that homeopathy can necessarily do better. In a way its advantage is that it does not need a diagnosis to justify treatment. It takes the manifestation of the illness at its face value as a legitimate indication of need and a sufficient indication for the homeopathic response to that need. In this sense we can trust to the body's own inherent wisdom to remedy the situation without the need for us to achieve a definitive explanation. If we find the right prescription this certainly happens. It is surprising how often changes take place on a psychological level, for example, without any discussion of the dynamics, which if we sought them through psychotherapy would require considerable insight gained at the cost of a great deal of time. Homeopathy may stimulate change in this unconscious way without the need for a conventional diagnostic rationale on which to base the treatment. Whatever the possibility of this, however, it does not absolve us from the responsibility of working out with the patient if not the best possible explanation of the illness at least the best possible interpretation, and in this the perspectives discussed here can be of value. In the first place such an interpretation is essential if the illness is to have some meaning for the patient; and it is this that many of us seek as well as a means of recovery. Secondly it is essential if the patient is to be able to make the changes in their life that will assist their recovery and promote their greater health and well-being in the future. The concept of an underlying and unifying state of disequilibrium seems to be helpful. It allows for the multifactorial evolution of the individual's present state of health and for its multifaceted presentation, but relates them to a coherent whole. This makes sense to patients who intuitively distrust the fragmentation that conventional medicine imposes by the 'separatist' approach to systems of the body, disorders and episodes of illness that has already been discussed. Homeopathy not only embraces this as a philosophical point of view, but bases its rationale of treatment upon it, in as much as particular perspectives indicate particular treatments.

REFERENCES

Balint M 1964 The doctor, his patient and the illness, 2nd edn. Pitman, London, ch 7

FURTHER READING

Clarke J 1924, 1925 Case taking, parts 1, 2 and 3. Homeopathic World 59(706): 295–300, 313–318; 60 (709): 12–16
Kunzli J 1974 How to take the case. Journal of the American Institute of Homeopathy 67(3): 165–168
Morrison R 1990, 1991 Methods of case analysis, parts 1, 2 and 3. Journal of the American Institute of Homeopathy 83(3): 63–71; 83(4): 118–125; 84(1): 20–26

5

Symptoms

THE INDIVIDUALITY OF SYMPTOMS

The idiosyncratic use of the term 'symptom' in homeopathy to include physical signs and even pathological states has been mentioned already. To most clinicians symptoms are patients' subjective experiences of their illnesses. In some disciplines the term may be restricted to those experiences that are recognized characteristics of a specific disorder leading to a diagnosis. This view provides an interesting comparison with homeopathy. There is similarity in the use of symptoms, common in all medicine of course, to establish a diagnosis, including in homeopathy the diagnosis of the prescription. There is also complete contrast in that symptoms are taken seriously in homeopathy *whether or not* they are recognized features of a previously known condition or of the known materia medica of any homeopathic medicines.

In fact the greatest contrast between the conventional and homeopathic use of symptoms is that in homeopathy the most valuable symptoms are those that are *not* typical of underlying pathology. In conventional medicine the reverse is true. The most useful clinical findings (symptoms, signs, test results) are those that are characteristic of the disorder, and hence most commonplace among patients who present with that disorder. In homeopathy the clinical features most commonly found in patients with a particular disorder, most characteristic of the disorder, are the least useful in determining the prescription. The first rule of symptomatology in homeopathy is that the value of symptoms, meaning all clinical findings, is directly proportional to their individuality. This is one of the essential principles described in Chapter 2 (p. 22). It cannot be emphasized too strongly. The most important symptoms are those that are characteristic of the patient and of the behaviour of the illness in that patient. These will most clearly define the similarity between the clinical picture in the patient and the characteristics of the medicine. The effective medicine will be the one in which this similarity is most complete.

The analogy between the process of the conventional differential diagnosis of the illness and the homeopathic differential diagnosis of the prescription breaks down at this point. The first depends on identifying the common manifestations of the illness in the patient, the second on identifying those that are not common to most patients but most individual to this particular patient (Fig. 5.1).

For this reason the pathological findings and physical signs are likely to be least useful in individualizing the prescription. The pathology of any disease or syndrome varies little from patient to patient. It may differ in location or extent, involve different organisms, show different levels of abnormality in the blood and so on. These will be of relevance to the homeopathic prescription and may have to be a feature of the prescription. But because they will be found in the materia medica of many homeopathic medicines that include that pathology they will not by themselves identify the one prescription that the patient needs. Physical signs may vary more than pathological findings between patients with the same illness. The location and character of abnormal breath sounds may differ to a certain extent in different patients with bronchitis. The sounds may be differently affected by deep breathing, coughing or posture. But these differences will not go far in discriminating between the number of possible medicines, only one of which will meet the need of the individual patient.

The features of an illness that most clearly define its character in the individual are the subjective symptoms – their precise detail, the pattern that they form collectively (their picture or totality) and, most importantly, their behaviour.

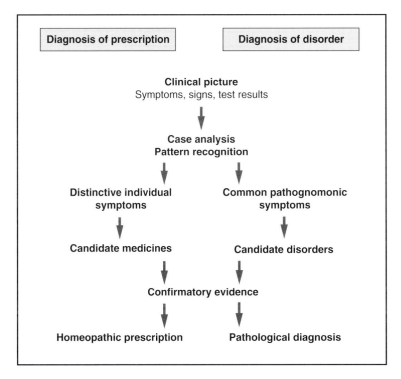

Figure 5.1 'Differential diagnosis' in homeopathy uses the most distinctively individual symptoms rather than those most commonly associated with the disorder.

MODALITIES

The ways in which symptoms are influenced by commonplace events or activities of everyday life comprise their most individual features. Factors that may influence their behaviour range from the time of day and the weather, through physical activities and body functions to emotional states and social circumstances. These modifying factors are known as 'modalities'.

Any one symptom may have a number of modalities. The more modalities a symptom possesses the more precisely it is defined, and the more precisely it is defined the more precisely it is likely to be matched to the drug picture of a particular medicine. There are 10 medicines listed for left-sided sore throat, 17 for sore throat that is worse in the morning (4 on waking), 8 that are aggravated by warm drinks and 19 that have pain extending to the ear on swallowing. 43 medicines share one or more of these characteristics, but only one, Lachesis, has a left-sided sore throat worse on waking in the morning that is aggravated by warm drinks and spreads to the ear on swallowing. It may seem extravagantly hard work to select the prescription in this case if an aspirin gargle would do, and indeed it might be so, but it is a familiar scenario and makes the point. And if the problem were recurrent then aspirin gargles would not be the answer.

Of course, modalities are a familiar part of conventional diagnosis – breathlessness when lying down, heartburn when stooping, morning stiffness and so on. The difference between the conventional and homeopathic approach is one of degree, not of kind. What is of surpassing interest is the significance of these individual differences. Why do two patients with the same sore throat, in the sense that they may share the same epidemic cause and onset, have different pain reactions to hot and cold drinks? What does it mean in terms of neuropeptide response, in terms of their constitutional disposition and susceptibility to other illness, in terms of the stimulus the body may need to reinforce its self-regulating response? That these differences do define the specific need, the particular dynamics of the healing process in the individual, is evident in the effects of the medicines specifically indicated by them. If, that is, we are to accept their efficacy. Even if we do not, the other questions remain pertinent. What do these differences mean? This is the kind of question that recurs whatever aspect we examine of the phenomenon of illness and healing that homeopathy demonstrates. (See also Ch. 11, p. 202, Significant differences.)

The most difficult patients to treat are those whose symptoms are few and commonplace, particularly if they lack modalities. Fortunately this is not often the case, and modalities can be particularly useful when a patient has difficulty describing the precise nature of symptoms. The character of pain, for example, can be difficult to describe, but the behaviour of the pain in response to modifying factors is usually easy. A patient may be vague as to whether a pain is burning or raw or pricking, but is likely to know when it hurts and what makes it hurt.

TYPES OF SYMPTOM

Three types of symptom are distinguished: local or particular, general and mental. The particular symptoms are the subject matter of the close-up view described in the last chapter. They are the particular and localized problem presented by the patient – usually a specific complaint referred to a specific part or system of the body. General symptoms, not surprisingly, concern the general physical condition and body functions associated with the presenting complaint: body temperature, thirst, appetite, bowel and bladder function, menstruation, sweat, sleep, etc. Mental symptoms might of course be the 'local' symptoms if the presenting problem is the mental state of the patient. When this is not the case they refer to the state of mind of the patient associated with the presenting symptoms. They can involve consciousness, intellect, mood or emotions. Modalities apply to all three types of symptom, and symptoms themselves can act as modalities. Mental states can act as modalities to physical symptoms (e.g. 'The pain is worse if I get angry'). Physical symptoms can act as modalities to mental symptoms (e.g. 'She gets very bad-tempered when she starts to get wheezy'), and to other physical symptoms (an obvious example would be urinary incontinence aggravated by a cough).

One value of this classification of symptoms is to make it easier to be systematic in obtaining a complete clinical picture. Another is said to be their relative importance when analysing the case. This is open to debate, but it is held that mental symptoms have the highest importance, general symptoms the next and local symptoms the least: the so-called 'hierarchy of symptoms'. This is consistent with the view that mental symptoms are of similarly greater significance for the individuality of the patient's condition and their level of well-being. A third reason for distinguishing the three types of symptom is the principle that a combination of at least one of each in the clinical picture is necessary to define the similimum – the best-matched prescription. This is a useful rule of thumb, but need not be followed slavishly. It is the minimalist approach to the concept of the totality of symptoms.

THE TOTALITY OF SYMPTOMS

It is the totality of symptoms that ensures the uniquely individual character of the clinical picture. It encompasses everything that is going on in the patient in the course of the current illness – pathological states, physical signs, subjective symptoms; local, general and mental features; and all modalities.

Multiple symptoms

The totality may consist only of the features of the presenting complaint. In an acute illness or injury this will probably be the case. In chronic illness it is rarely so, and where one disorder is compounded by another the possible permutations of individual symptomatology increase enormously. Many patients who seek homeopathy do have multiple symptomatology. This can of course provide plenty of material from which to identify the relevant medicine. But when there are symptoms in profusion it becomes increasingly difficult to see the wood for the trees. Any general practitioner will be familiar with this problem and its 'heart sink' potential. It can create as much despair for the homeopath if the key symptoms are not carefully identified. The selection of key symptoms as indications for the prescription is dealt with in the following sections.

Where there are multiple symptoms the totality is more than the sum of its parts. The symptom cluster for each separate complaint presented by the patient may consist of its own local, general and mental features and their modalities. Each of these clusters may suggest the same similimum, the one specific medicine. But it is possible that analysed separately each could suggest a different hierarchy of medicines, the hierarchy being the order of similarity of the possible medicines indicated by that particular symptom cluster. Thus a patient with headache, irritable bowel and a skin eruption may present a cluster of symptoms for each, each of which matches a different group of possible medicines. Or the groups appropriate to each symptom cluster may include some of the same medicines but in different orders of similarity. The solution to this confusing or contradictory state of affairs is to identify the common features of each cluster of symptoms that represent a consistent view of the whole. These common features will usually be found to transcend the differences between the parts, the separate symptom clusters. They may also fit in with one of the wider perspectives of the patient that have been discussed. This might be the constitutional picture, based on the characteristics of the person rather than the illness alone (see Ch. 6), or the historical view, which describes the evolution of the illness and its contributory factors

SELECTING AND EVALUATING SYMPTOMS
Recording the symptoms

Because it is so obvious a fact it seems almost impertinent to point out that nothing in the case history will be of value unless it is carefully and accurately elicited in the first place. This is equally true and equally obvious whatever medical discipline we work in. Nevertheless we are probably more likely to mistake the correct diagnosis or prescription because we have not elicited, recognized or understood some key piece of information when taking the case history than for any other reason. This is not always our fault. It may indeed result from lack of attention but it may be that the patient has not divulged the information, by chance, through forgetfulness or even deliberately. This is why, however much we allow and encourage a spontaneous account of things from the patient, we must also be systematic. Unless the key information is clearly and readily available we must leave no stone unturned to find it.

There are two provisos to this statement. First, we have to remember the temptation to find the 'pattern with which we are familiar' or that particularly interests us at the time. We have all experienced the surprisingly high incidence of conditions or symptom pictures that we have just learned about in the days following the lecture or after reading the book. The second proviso is that we must maintain a high level of courtesy towards the patient and turn each stone with care and sensitivity, or wait for a more opportune moment. A callous, clumsy or untimely enquiry may inhibit a true understanding of the matter as much as if we had not enquired in the first place. Nevertheless we must, with due sensitivity, be prepared to enquire into any facet of a patient's life if it will help us and the patient to do so. We may often feel embarrassed, for example, to ask about patients' sex lives – embarrassed for ourselves as well as them. But this can be a highly individual and distinctive aspect of a patient's physical, general and emotional state. It may provide a key piece of the jigsaw, whether it concerns the time in the menstrual cycle when a woman's libido is highest, or to do with feelings about sex, or past sexual experiences, or a history of venereal disease.

Presenting and incidental symptoms

The relative significance of presenting symptoms and incidental symptoms has been touched upon already. Presenting symptoms may be of great importance because they are what most intensely concern the patient. On the other hand they may be of relatively minor importance in the face of other coexisting problems. These may be given lesser priority by the patient because they think they are not a proper subject for homeopathy, or because they are already being treated and reasonably well controlled with conventional medicine. The presenting symptoms are of primary importance when they do represent the most pressing of the patient's concerns. Otherwise they should be evaluated alongside the other symptoms that are elicited in the course of our enquiry, which may be of greater consequence than those first presented in terms of both the patient's overall well-being and our goals of treatment.

Pathology

Two other threads from earlier sections need to be picked up again here. These concern the relative usefulness, or lack of it, of common features of the underlying pathology in the clinical picture, and the focus on pathology (the local, pathological prescription), which was described as part of the close-up view. Features of the pathology that are common to all patients with a particular disorder are not as a rule useful for *individualizing* the clinical picture. By definition, only those features that are characteristic of the way the disorder is expressed in the individual patient are useful for that purpose. Pathological features are used as indications, however, and pathological prescriptions can be very effective.

A case study

At this point I want to quote at some length a case study that demonstrates particularly clearly some of the issues that have been presented so far (Sommermann 1992). It focuses on the role of the pathology and the totality in the clinical picture, and on the contrast between the pathological and the individual view of the patient, and on the relationship between them.

The case concerns a 42-year-old Vietnam war veteran with non-Hodgkin's lymphoma induced by exposure to Agent Orange. He had received 4 months' chemotherapy, interrupted for 3 months prior to starting homeopathy because of his extreme anxiety at having to travel from the country into the city for treatment. His severe chronic anxiety, following his experiences in Vietnam, was the dominant feature of his clinical picture alongside the pathological features of the lymphoma. The clinical features of this included lymphadenopathy and, most conspicuously, extreme splenomegaly, about 10 times the normal size.

The totality of the symptoms, in which his mental state predominated, and the constitutional characteristics of the man strongly indicated a particular medicine, Argenticum nitricum (Arg. n.), but its materia medica does not include enlargement of the spleen (Box 5.1). This is not just a main pathological feature of the disease but a literally huge feature of the clinical picture and a source of great discomfort to the patient. Its size had been reduced by chemotherapy but it had enlarged again since, and splenectomy was being recommended. None of the other medicines suggested by the totality covered the picture so convincingly as Arg. n., and some also did not include the pathology of the spleen. In his report the author writes: 'After I got to this point, I threw out the totality and looked at the case from the "pathology first" perspective. I do this when the pathology is very strong and I can't see a (medicine) that covers the whole case. After all, this man's spleen is huge—it hangs down to his navel.' He investigated the materia medica of all the medicines associated with enlargement of the spleen. He immediately chose Ceanothus. This is a 'small remedy', a homeopathic medicine whose known materia medica does not include a variety of symptoms, but it is the only small remedy in 'bold type' (indicating a very strong association) listed for enlarged spleen. Ceanothus Americanus was introduced into homeopathy by an English physician James Compton Burnett in 1879 (Burnett 1900, Tyler 1952). Boericke's materia medica says of it: 'This (medicine) seems to possess a specific relation to the spleen – enormous enlargement of the spleen – Splenitis –

Leukaemia' (Boericke 1927). The author writes, 'As far as the pathology goes, this (medicine) fits the bill perfectly'. He later quotes Burnett as stating that 'organopathy' is correctly used only when a similimum that covers the totality and the pathology cannot be found.

Box 5.1 Lymphoma patient: Argentum nitricum symptoms and characteristics

Complaints from fright **Fear of being alone** *Fear of high places* *Fear of crowds* *Fear of public places* Fear of crossing bridges **Complaints from anticipation**

Anxious feeling in stomach   Nightmares   *Anxious restlessness in bed*

Hyperventilation   Libido diminished   *Vertigo in high places*

Pain in stomach + *Aggravated by alcohol*

PHYSICAL CONSTITUTION: *Warm blooded, feels the heat*   **Thirsty**

PERSONALITY (not graded):   Friendly, straightforward, open, easy to get to know, emotional

---

Repertory grading of symptoms (see p. 98) is shown by standard use of type:
Bold = Grade 3, *Italic* = Grade 2, Plain = Grade 1.

Treatment with Ceanothus was 12C (centesimal dilution) daily until there was evidence of a proving (increase in Ceanothus features following continuous repetition of the dose), then Ceanothus 30C every 2 weeks. This produced a striking improvement in the clinical features of the lymphoma, which was maintained at the last reported follow-up a year later. Meanwhile, however, the clinical picture had changed. Six months after improvement in his lymphoma had been achieved he expressed a desire to see a psychiatrist because of his anxiety. He now revealed intense symptoms of Arg. n., including a craving for sweets and salt and persistent conjunctivitis. He was given Arg. n. and improved greatly within 2 weeks. A further 6 months later (last reported follow-up) he announced himself as feeling 95% better. The whole case study covers a 19-month period.

This case demonstrates the following features:

- the close-up and the wide-angle views of the patient – that is, the pathology and the totality
- their coexistence as two layers of the illness
- the importance of the pathology in this case, and its dominance of the clinical picture
- the choice of the pathological prescription at the expense of the totality because of the essential importance of the pathology and the absence of an appropriate totality
- the emergence of the more fundamental psychological layer after the resolution of the pathology, and its subsequent response to the appropriate similimum.

One other point is worth mentioning. In the course of treatment a number of observations were made of the action of Ceanothus on the patient, some from its therapeutic effects, some from the provings. Some of these observations of Ceanothus symptoms were new; they were not previously known to be associated with Ceanothus. If they are corroborated in other patients treated with Ceanothus, they will, in time, earn a legitimate place in its materia medica. This is an example of the development of the materia medica through clinical experience.

Eliminating symptoms

The case also illustrates another approach to the use of symptoms as indications. This is the role of the eliminating symptom. Here the practitioner decided that the enlargement of the spleen was so dominant a feature of the case that it must be represented in the clinical picture on which he prescribed, and hence be a feature of the materia medica of his chosen medicine. Other medicines that might have represented the similimum were eliminated because they did not cover the spleen.

Any type of symptom may be used as an eliminating symptom. The criterion for its use is that it must be such a vivid and essential feature of the clinical picture that no medicine that does not include it in its repertoire can possibly be considered similar. If such a symptom can be identified it simplifies the selection of the best medicine by excluding those that match much of the totality but not the key symptom. In the case study no medicine that approximated to the totality also covered the key symptom. This led to the choice of a pathological prescription that captured it precisely rather than one based on the totality.

A problem here is the fact that the materia medica of some, perhaps many, medicines is not necessarily complete. Nevertheless, the use of eliminating symptoms is a valuable technique if applied with judgement and discretion.

Criteria of a 'good symptom'

The word that best sums up for me the characteristics of a symptom that we may use with confidence to select the correct homeopathic medicine is 'vivid'. The symptoms that most vividly express the patient's experience of the illness are most likely to lead to the right prescription. The characteristics that make a symptom most vivid are spontaneity, clarity, intensity and individuality.

The value of information volunteered spontaneously by the patient has been mentioned already. There can also be a quality of spontaneity about the way a patient responds to a prompt or an enquiry. This can sometimes lead to such a lively response that it has much of the quality of a wholly spontaneous remark. Where a symptom is presented with this kind of energy I am inclined to treat it as spontaneous even if it is not wholly volunteered. The quality of clarity is self-explanatory. Many symptoms are described quite vaguely, and cannot be better defined, even with help (paraphrase, etc.). A symptom that is clearly presented is likely to have had considerable impact on the patient: to have been experienced vividly and so vividly expressed. The strength or intensity of the symptom may include its severity or magnitude (the enormous spleen), or some similar aspect of its impact upon the patient (disgust, terror, etc.). This is likely to be reflected in the emphasis or intensity with which it is described.

The importance of the individuality of the symptoms has been continually stressed. Instead of being dismayed, as one may be in conventional medicine, by the description of a symptom that we have never before heard of, and that fits absolutely no pattern with which we are familiar, the homeopath should be delighted. It is likely to be vividly expressive of the individual illness and a key indication for the prescription. Despite its unfamiliarity it is surprisingly likely to be recorded in the literature of some homeopathic medicine. And now that computers give us the ability to search the whole literature for particular groups of words in seconds, there is a real possibility of finding it. If there really is no previous record of a symptom in the literature, or very few records of it, then this imposes a responsibility on us to note its apparent association with the medicine that effectively remedies it (if that is achieved) as a possible addition to its materia medica.

Strange, rare and peculiar symptoms

The symptoms traditionally accorded the highest esteem for their individuality are described as 'strange, rare and peculiar'. A strange symptom would be the sensation that a ball bearing is rolling around inside the eyeball. It would also be rare. It would be peculiar if the eyeball had been removed surgically. A rare symptom would be an aversion to chocolate before menstruation. It is not strange, because such changes in tastes for food are commonplace, nor is such a change peculiar in association with hormone changes. But it is extremely rare because if a woman experiences a change of taste for chocolate in midcycle or before her period it is virtually always a craving. The latter is so common a feature of the premenstrual syndrome (PMS) that it is no use as an individualizing symptom. After many years of special interest in PMS I can recall only one patient who actually went off chocolate. Unfortunately no homeopathic medicine is yet associated with this change, as far as I know.

Peculiar symptoms are not necessarily strange in nature but are an anomaly in the context of the patient's other attributes or symptoms. For a patient who is placid in all respects, but quickly enraged in one particular circumstance, that reaction and its modality, the factor responsible, would be valuably peculiar. Such symptoms are often paradoxical; breathlessness relieved by motion is an example. The medicine Ferrum, derived from metallic iron, is uniquely associated with breathlessness *relieved* by motion and talking.

This section is a personal interpretation of these concepts, which are not explicitly defined with clear authority in any source I know of. Hahnemann refers to them quite generally in paragraph 153 of his original treatise, the Organon: 'in this search for a homeopathic specific remedy . . . the more striking, singular, uncommon and peculiar (characteristic) signs and symptoms . . . are chiefly and most solely to be kept in view; for it is more particularly these that very similar ones in the list of symptoms of the selected medicine must correspond to, in order to constitute it the most suitable for effecting the cure' (Hahnemann & Dudgeon 1982).

These facets of 'strange, rare and peculiar' are teased out in this way to demonstrate the specially individualizing properties of such symptoms. In effect, though, the concept can be taken as a collective phase for any features that are most vividly and idiosyncratically distinctive of patients' unique experience of their illnesses.

Such characteristics do not need to be presented by the patients themselves. My first encounter with such a symptom was during a series of consultations with a 13-year-old boy with psoriasis in general practice. Building up a clinical picture cumulatively from one consultation to the next, and so far unavailingly, I got round to asking whether he was tidy. 'My God', said his mother, 'He's so tidy he drives me mad! ' Her outcry had all the quality of spontaneity, and absolute clarity. It also revealed a 'symptom' of great intensity, and in a 13-year-old boy markedly strange, rare and peculiar. The prescription of Arsenicum suddenly became obvious; and it proved effective.

Complete symptoms

A symptom will be most vivid and therefore most useful if all its potential characteristics are fully described. A symptom may have the following four facets: general nature of the symptom (pain; eruption), detailed character (pain – throbbing; eruption – moist, crusty, itching), location (pain – left temple, radiating to left eye; eruption – behind the ears), and behaviour or modalities (pain – worse on lying down, worse on coughing, better with pressure; eruption – worse when anxious, better by the seaside). A complete symptom is one that has all its available characteristics described. Some symptoms will not have all four facets. Difficulty in breathing, for instance, will not have a site. On the other hand some symptoms have facets that would not always be thought about. Anxiety, for example, can be felt in various locations. Some facets will involve several descriptors; the example of the eruption had three descriptive details, and the pain in the temple three modalities. Separate descriptors of detail might have separate modalities; the itching of the eruption might be worse at night in bed.

The more complete the symptom and the fuller the description of each facet, the more precise the identity of the similar medicine is likely to be.

Concomitant symptoms

These are symptoms that occur at the same time as the primary symptoms; they are simultaneous or directly associated in time – immediately, or at a precise interval before or after. Incidental symptoms may occur concurrently or intercurrently and are part of the patient's current clinical picture, but they do not have a direct association with the primary symptom. Itching eyes, puffy lids and sneezing might be concomitant symptoms in hay fever because they are directly associated with one another and occur simultaneously. They would not be especially useful in identifying the prescription, however, because they are very commonplace concomitants. A patient might present with a complaint of headache and report in passing that they often feel hungry, or that they sometimes pass a profuse amount of urine. These symptoms are incidental to the main complaint of headache. But if the patient always feels hungry (a general symptom) during a headache, or passes copious urine as or just after their headache resolves, these are concomitant symptoms. Concomitant symptoms that are not commonly associated with the primary symptom are of particular value in identifying the correct medicine (Box 5.2). We might add concomitants as another possible facet of a complete symptom.

Two instances of the problem of 'repertory language' arise from these examples. Some repertories express hunger only as 'appetite increased'. More recent editions attach hunger as a synonym, but increased appetite is not necessarily associated with hunger. Profuse urination is shown as ameliorating the headache. What most patients actually describe is profuse urination accompanying or following the relief of the headache. A causal association between the two may be speculative. Patients have not told me that their headache goes if they can manage to pass a lot of water. On the other hand, patients do say that if they don't drink enough they get headaches.

Box 5.2 Concomitant symptoms associated with headache*

Makes mistakes writing	Nux moschata
Weakness of memory	Belladonna
Trembling	Argentum nitricum
Unable to open eyes	*Tarentula*
Acute sense of smell	**Phosphorus**
Coldness of the face	*Carbo vegetabilis* Arsenicum
	Ipecacuanha
Burning pain in stomach	Sanguinaria
Scanty urine during, copious after	Sanguinaria Glycyrrhiza
Sexual desire increased	Sepia
Palpitations	*Spigelia* Argentum nitricum(+ 4)
Coldness of foot (postmenstrual headache)	*Ferrum*
Weakness of hand and/or foot	Oleum animale

*Symptoms specific to single or very few medicines, showing repertory grades.

These are semantic problems for the homeopathic literature, but they are also fascinating examples of the opportunities for natural history and the possible physiological insights that homeopathy offers.

Summary

The most valuable symptoms for the differential diagnosis of the homeopathic medicine are those that are most complete in their description and that most vividly express the individual character of the illness. These symptoms combine to form a totality of symptoms, which may comprise a number of separate complaints. The complete clinical picture that they represent is usually the best basis for selecting the prescription. A more circumscribed view of the case, even a single pathological feature, may, however, sometimes be used. This is justified by the overwhelming significance of the particular feature, especially if the totality does not adequately encompass it.

GRADING OF SYMPTOMS

The purpose of grading symptoms is to assist in the selection of those that will provide the key indications for the chosen medicine. The selection of symptoms will be successful only if they are elicited and recorded thoroughly, carefully and perceptively in the first place. Similarly, their grading will have any meaning and value only if their significance has been properly assessed. The value of this assessment will in turn be lost if it is not recorded in the notes and readily available when the case comes to be analysed.

Grading of symptoms is a common feature of the repertories. The grades are represented by the type in which the names of the medicines are printed. Nowadays four grades are often used: bold capitals for the highest, bold lower case for the next, italic for the next and plain type for the lowest grade. This formalism denotes the range from a highest grade medicine, in which the symptom or characteristic is vividly and indisputably represented, down to those in which it has been observed but with no great intensity or high degree of corroboration. The repertory grades are supposed to represent the frequency with which the symptom has been caused by the medicine in provings and cured by it in clinical practice. The strictness and consistency with which these criteria are applied is open to question. The so-called 'small remedies', those that have few known symptoms in their materia medica, and the 'plain type' medicines in the repertories, can have dramatic effects that extend beyond their familiar repertoire. It is often said that there are no small remedies, only little known ones. The grading in the repertories needs to be interpreted flexibly or we will ignore many useful medicines because of their lowly grade.

The grading of symptoms in the patient, however, need be subject to no such uncertainty if we are disciplined in our approach. As in the repertories, four grades may be useful. The top grade, usually marked '4' rather than '1', is a definitive indication for the chosen medicine. It is effectively an eliminating symptom. The chosen medicine *must* include it in its materia medica and with similar intensity. Grade 3 is strongly indicative. Grade 2 symptoms will probably feature in the chosen medicine but are negotiable. Grade 1 symptoms are not at all definitive, but may provide corroboration. They are only just more interesting than ungraded symptoms, which are commonplace and/or vague.

Grade 4 would be the tidiness of the boy with psoriasis. This is really a constitutional characteristic rather than a symptom (see next chapter), but definitely grade 4. Pushing for grade 4, but certainly grade 3, would be the examples of concomitant symptoms. A strong, clear, complete symptom such as burning epigastric pain after eating, radiating to the back and relieved by belching (Carbo vegetabilis) would be a good grade 3. Less vivid, more poorly described and more commonplace symptoms are progressively grades 2 and 1. Occasional mild burning epigastric pain after eating might make grade 1, but is almost too commonplace a dyspeptic symptom to be helpful.

The allocation of grades becomes clearer with experience and can really only be judged by the way the symptom is actually expressed by the patient. No description of a scale of grades like this can be more than a rule of thumb, but the principle and the discipline of grading symptoms are important. Without it our case analysis will be hit and miss, and it will be difficult to recall the justification for the prescription later.

The grading of symptoms interacts with another axis of evaluation, which is the hierarchy of symptoms mentioned earlier in which mental symptoms (state of mind, intellectual performance, mood, emotions) have the greatest importance, general symptoms the next and local symptoms the least. The hierarchy would really only apply if otherwise equally strong symptoms were pointing to different choices of medicine and their relative importance had to be established. On this basis a case analysis would favour the one in which the mental symptoms were best represented. It is probably better to regard this as just one perspective within which to evaluate symptoms. The overriding consideration is which combination of symptoms most vividly and faithfully expresses the disturbed equilibrium of the patient.

Several of the points discussed in this and adjacent chapters are illustrated in the case study (Box 5.3).

RECURRING THEMES

It may often happen that certain characteristics of symptoms emerge as recurring themes in the case history. These themes may embrace local, general or mental symptoms. For example, all sensations may be burning – the pain, discharges, eruptions, hot feet, chilblains, etc.; or all symptoms may be one sided – left-sided headaches, tennis elbow, abdominal pain, sciatica,

---

Box 5.3   Case analysis

Mr H. A. (aged 64) was referred for treatment of reflux oesophagitis of 5 years' duration, preceded by many years of indigestion. In addition he suffered from irritable bowel symptoms and a barium enema had revealed mild diverticulitis. Two distinctive patterns of symptoms were described and are depicted in Figure 5.2A and B. The figure is derived from the printout of a computer analysis (repertorization) of the key features (CARA 1996). Each part of the figure shows a number of medicines whose materia medica includes the selected symptoms. The grade with which the symptom is represented by each medicine is shown in the squares of the grid. The importance of each symptom in the patient's clinical picture is shown to the far left of the symptom rubric. Each symptom rubric shows the source of the data (the name of the repertory), then the site or type of the symptom, then the symptom detail. The symbol ' < ' means 'made worse by'.

No single medicine is identified with every key symptom and groups of medicines that correspond best to each set of symptoms differ. Two medicines occur in each group: Causticum and Phosphorus. Figure 5.2C shows a 'strange, rare and peculiar' symptom – frequent waking at midnight with such a start that the patient is jerked out of bed – and a number of 'constitutional' characteristics. Overall, Causticum is best represented, and when the analysis is applied to the most distinctly individual symptoms (Fig. 5.2D) the choice of Causticum is even more strongly emphasized. The 'total weighted score' shows the additional emphasis provided by the relative rarity with which the particular symptom is found in the materia medica. The fewer medicines that include it, the greater is the emphasis.

Causticum is the medicine whose materia medica or 'drug picture' is most like the 'clinical picture'. This is the 'similimum', the medicine whose characteristics are most similar to the individual presentation of the totality of symptoms, the whole pattern of disorder in this patient.

This choice must not be made on the basis of this repertory analysis of the case alone. It has to be corroborated by the clinician's more intimate knowledge of the patient and of the materia medica. Alternatively, additional materia medica study may be needed to refine or confirm the repertorization, which can never do more than suggest the most likely candidate medicines. The correct choice will often *not* be the medicine at the top of the list.

---

phlebitis, etc. There may be a tendency to excess – loquacity, perspiration, skin excrescences, heavy or prolonged menstruation. There may be a tendency to coldness – emotional, internal, or of the extremities. There may be such a pervasive pattern in these themes that it must be represented in the medicine, like an eliminating symptom; or the theme may have a symbolic, psychosomatic significance.

One patient expressed this clearly as she concluded a consultation about her watering eyes and vaginal discharge with the words, 'Oh dear, I seem to be weeping at both ends'. Her

						K		
	C	N U			N A		
	A P U		B L	A L	P		
	U U X	B R	Y T	I	H		
	S L -	R Y	- -	-	O		
	T S V	Y C	M C	S			

CARA chart, (3) Printed:11/1/97 5:06:47 p.m.
Analysis type: Totality

Remedy filters
Polychrest: Yes
Frequent: Yes
Small: Yes
Nosodes: Yes
Remedy class: All
Remedy family: All
Miasmas: All

Rubric filters
Rubric weightings: Yes
Stress significance: Yes
Emphasise SRP: No
Emphasise small: No

	CAUST	NUX-V	PULS	BRY	LYC	NAT-M	KALI-C	PHOS
Total (weighted) score	15	15	14	12	12	12	9	9
Total rubrics covered	5	3	5	3	4	3	4	5
Total grades scored	9	9	9	7	9	7	5	8
1 Combined Kent Stomach **HEARTBURN**	2	3	3	2	3	2	2	2
1 Combined Kent Stomach **ERUCTATIONS, ACRID**	2		2		3			1
1 Combined Kent Chest **PAIN, STERNUM, BEHIND**								2
1 Combined Kent Chest **PAIN, BURNING, STERNUM, UNDER**								2
2 Combined Synthetic Generals **FOOD, FARINACEOUS FOOD**	2	3	1	2	1	3	1	
2 Combined Synthetic Generals **FOOD, BREAD**	2	3	2	3	2	2	1	1
3 Murphy Generals **TIME, NIGHT 3 a.m. TO 4 a.m.**	1		1				1	

Figure 5.2A

Figure 5.2 Details of case analysis described in Box 5.3. A: Symptoms of reflux oesophagitis. B: Symptoms of irritable bowel and diverticulitis. C: Strange, rare and peculiar (SRP) symptoms and constitutional features. D: Most distinctively individual symptoms.

CARA chart, (3) Printed:11/1/97 5:25:21 p.m.						
Analysis type: Totality						

Remedy filters		**Rubric filters**	
Polychrest:	Yes	Rubric weightings:	Yes
Frequent:	Yes	Stress significance:	Yes
Small:	Yes	Emphasise SRP:	No
Nosodes:	Yes	Emphasise small:	No
Remedy class:	All		
Remedy family:	All		
Miasmas:	All		

				CAUST	SULPH	ALOE	PHOS	ARG-N	ZINC	BRY	COLOC
		Total (weighted) score		25	20	19	18	14	14	13	13
		Total rubrics covered		7	5	5	6	4	6	5	5
		Total grades scored		13	12	14	12	8	8	10	9
2	Combined Kent	Abdomen	DISTENSION EVENING	1		2			1	2	
1	Combined Kent	Rectum	DIARRHOEA MORNING		2	3	3	2	2	3	2
2	Combined Kent	Rectum	URGING, BREAKFAST, AFTER								
1	Combined Kent	Rectum	URGING (IN GENERAL)	1	2	3	2	2	1	2	2
1	Combined Kent	Rectum	INVOLUNTARY, STOOL	2	3	3	3	1	1	2	2
3	Combined Kent	Rectum	FLATUS, INVOLUNTARY				1				
3	Combined Kent	Rectum	FLATUS, LOUD	3	3		1	3	2		1
2	Combined Kent	Rectum	SPASMS, IN	2							
2	Combined Kent	Rectum	PAIN (IN GENERAL)	3	2	3	2		1	1	2
1	Combined Kent	Rectum	PAIN, GRIPPING								
1	Murphy	Stool	MUCUS, COVERED WITH MUCUS	1							

Figure 5.2B

CARA chart, (3) Printed:11/1/97 5:36:37 p.m.
Analysis type: Totality

Remedy filters		Rubric filters	
Polychrest:	Yes	Rubric weightings:	Yes
Frequent:	Yes	Stress significance:	Yes
Small:	Yes	Emphasise SRP:	No
Nosodes:	Yes	Emphasise small:	No
Remedy class:	All		
Remedy family:	All		
Miasmas:	All		

			CAUST	CARS	KALI-ONC	MIRC	META-RCM	NAUX-MV	NUX-V	PHOS
		Total (weighted) score	21	18	12	12	12	12	12	12
		Total rubrics covered	4	5	2	3	3	4	4	3
		Total grades scored	9	9	5	5	6	7	5	5
3 Murphy	Sleep	STARTLED, DURING/ FROM SLEEP	3	2	2	2	2	2	2	2
2 Murphy	Generals	TIME, MIDNIGHT	2	2	3	1		1	1	1
1 Combined Synthetic	Generals	FOOD, FARINACEOUS FOOD DESIRE						2		
1 Combined Synthetic	Generals	FOOD, BREAD DESIRE		2			2	2		
2 Combined Synthetic	Mentals	CARES, RELATIVES, ABOUT	2	1						
2 Combined Synthetic	Generals	FOOD, SWEETS AVERSION	2	2		2	2		1	2
2 Combined Synthetic	Mentals	INJUSTICE, CANNOT SUPPORT							1	1

Figure 5.2C

CARA chart, (3) Printed:11/1/97 5:49:06 p.m.
Analysis type: Totality

Remedy filters   **Rubric filters**
Polychrest: Yes   Rubric weightings: Yes
Frequent: Yes   Stress significance: Yes
Small: Yes   Emphasise SRP: No
Nosodes: Yes   Emphasise small: No
Remedy class: All
Remedy family: All
Miasmas: All

				CAUST	PULS	BRY	SULPH	ZINC	NAT-S	NAT-M	GRAPH
			Total (weighted) score	140	72	68	57	52	49	48	44
			Total rubrics covered	12	7	6	8	9	3	7	4
			Total grades scored	25	16	11	15	13	8	12	9
1	Combined Kent	Stomach	HEARTBURN	2	3	2	2	2	2	2	2
2	Combined Synthetic	Generals	FOOD, FARINACEOUS FOOD <	2	3	2	1		3	3	
2	Combined Synthetic	Generals	FOOD, BREAD <	2	3	3	2	2		2	
2	Combined Kent	Abdomen	DISTENSION EVENING	1		2	2	1		1	
3	Murphy	Generals	TIME, NIGHT 3 a.m. TO 4 a.m.	1							
2	Combined Kent	Rectum	URGING, BREAKFAST, AFTER								
3	Combined Kent	Rectum	FLATUS, INVOLUNTARY								
3	Combined Kent	Rectum	FLATUS, LOUD	3				2	3		
2	Combined Kent	Rectums	SPASMS, IN	2							
2	Combined Kent	Rectum	PAIN (IN GENERAL)	3	3	1	3	1		1	3
3	Murphy	Sleep	STARTLED, DURING/FROM SLEEP	3	2	1	2	1		2	1
2	Murphy	Generals	TIME, MIDNIGHT	3	2		1	1		1	
2	Combined Synthetic	Mentals	CARES, RELATIVES, ABOUT	2				1			
2	Combined Synthetic	Generals	FOOD, SWEETS AVERSION	2	1		2	2			3
2	Combined Synthetic	Mentals	INJUSTICE, CANNOT SUPPORT								

Figure 5.2D

unresolved grief at her mother's death and other hurts had emerged during the consultation, and her words provided the motif for the clinical picture and its evolution. This is a nice example of the importance of paying attention to the words that patients use to express their problems and the possible levels of meaning, and that of providing the opportunity to say such things. Both have their own therapeutic action irrespective of the understanding of the problem that they provide.

Recurring themes within the materia medica of a particular medicine or a patient's history are sometimes described as their 'essence'.

SYMPTOMS FROM THE PAST

A fascinating phenomenon that may be observed during the course of homeopathic treatment is the transient return of symptoms that the patient had experienced in the past: symptoms that appeared to have been resolved, but that were apparently only dormant. The disorder they represented may have been entirely different from the current illness and of no apparent relevance to the current clinical picture. The re-emergence of the symptoms as part of the process of recovery from the current illness implies quite the reverse – that there is indeed a connection. It suggests that the condition of which they were an earlier manifestation was part of a continuing process; that is, it was an aspect of an underlying disequilibrium which is also the cause of the present disorder. It suggests that the healing process, acting at this fundamental level, proceeds by working out the unresolved disorder that was a part of this underlying pattern in the past. It reveals the past illness as part of an evolutionary process from which the present illness has arisen, and which is being rewound and replayed as on a video or tape recorder as healing proceeds.

The most dramatic example of this in my own experience occurred in a woman in her fifties who was being treated for indigestion. During the response to treatment she experienced the recurrence of a quite specific and very distressing symptom from her early teenage years. At that time she had suffered a psychotic breakdown following the discovery that she was an adopted child. The episode had been managed chiefly with psychotropic drugs, and no particular attention was paid to the psychodynamics. One of the symptoms had been that when she looked in the mirror she was unable to recognize the face that she saw. It was this symptom that recurred during treatment. Not surprisingly it caused considerable distress. It was also completely unforeseen, because although the past events and illness had been mentioned during the case history the symptomatology of that episode had not been discussed. Also, at that time in my homeopathic career I was not experienced enough to be alert to the possibilities of this unwinding of the evolutionary process.

This phenomenon is possibly the most remarkable and thought provoking that may be encountered in the practice of homeopathy. It is also alleged, though I cannot yet confidently confirm it from my own experience, that the phenomenon can include symptoms of disorders in the past history of the family. These are disorders that are not manifest clinically in the patient, or indeed detectable on investigation. An example would be the transient occurrence of thirst and polyuria in a patient with a family history of diabetes, in the absence of any other stigmata of the condition in themselves. Of course in this case there is the possibility that diabetes might become manifest in the patient at some stage. The possibility of a predisposition to a familial illness is also present even when no hereditary mechanism has yet been demonstrated. The interesting feature of this phenomenon is that it is transient, and the patient does not go on to develop the condition. The implication is that the underlying trait is exhibited during the healing process and resolved. We cannot know whether it would have become manifest later in the course of events if the homeopathic intervention had not been made.

SYMPTOMS THAT DO NOT FIT

Problems can be caused in case analysis by symptoms that do not fit the picture. The pattern of symptoms may clearly represent a recognizable drug picture with the exception of one or two possibly quite glaring exceptions. This should not necessarily undermine our confidence in the prevailing clinical picture provided its other features are valid, though we should take particular care to justify it. If we see a reproduction of the Mona Lisa wearing a modern earring, it remains in essence the Mona Lisa.

Two reasons have already been given why odd features may crop up in an otherwise consistent clinical picture. One is the appearance of symptoms that actually belong to another layer of the illness. The other is the possibility that the materia medica on which we are basing our similimum is incomplete, or even incorrect. A third reason may be our own ignorance of the possible variety of forms that a particular symptom may take in the relevant materia medica, or our too-rigid interpretation of the references to it. If we do not know that Pulsatilla patients can be obstinate as well as yielding we may stumble when we encounter this apparent anomaly. Similarly if we do not know that generally warm-blooded Pulsatilla can be chilly in an acute state, we may be puzzled. If we believe that Phosphorus patients are frightened of thunderstorms (a bold capitals repertory entry), we may be disconcerted by an apparent Phosphorus patient who enjoys them. The truth may be that Phosphorus patients are intensely stimulated by thunderstorms and react either with fear or excitement, or even both.

We have to remember, however, that we are dealing with patterns in patients that are actually unique. We treat many patients with the same major medicines. Each patient will present a unique permutation of the known features of that medicine together with some that are entirely individual. There can be no pattern that embraces every possible unique permutation of individual detail. Somewhere there is a Mona Lisa with an earring or a ptosis, or whatever. *The* Mona Lisa remains the similimum.

There is one further consideration. Contemporary homeopaths are devoting a great deal of effort and energy to exploring the 'small remedies' in greater depth and investigating the properties of substances that are new to the homeopathic repertoire. The scope for this process of extension and refinement of the materia medica is almost infinite. Any substance has the theoretical possibility of showing therapeutic potential when its homeopathic properties are investigated. The implication is that more precise similarity between clinical pictures whose similimum we think we can identify and newly or better defined medicines may become possible. This should in turn make more profound and complete therapeutic action by the medicines possible. This is something of a nightmare scenario because the therapeutic possibility would be accompanied by the added difficulty of finding this more precise similimum from an increasing multitude of possible medicines. This is a practical and philosophical problem for the future, but perhaps not the distant future (van der Zee 1996).

REFERENCES

Boericke W 1927 Pocket manual of homeopathic materia medica, 9th edn. Boericke and Runyon, Philadelphia, pp 184–185
Burnett J 1900 Diseases of the spleen and their remedies clinically illustrated. James Epps, London
CARA (2.6 for Windows) 1996. Miccant, West Bridgnorth
Hahnemann S, Dudgeon R 1982 Organon of medicine, 5th and 6th edns. Jain, New Delhi pp 95–96
Sommerman E 1992 Agent Orange-induced lymphoma. In: King S, Kipnis S, Scott C (eds) Proceedings of the 1992 professional case conference. International Foundation for Homeopathy, Seattle, pp 13–27
Tyler M 1952 Homeopathic Drug Pictures, 3rd edn. Health Science Press, Holsworthy, pp 231–235
van der Zee H 1996 Hopeless or hopelessly simple? Homeopathic Links 9: 62

FURTHER READING

Rieberer G 1995 Introduction to repertorisation. In: Foundation course in medical homeopathy. Royal London Homeopathic Hospital NHS Trust Academic Departments of Research and Education, London

6

Constitution

THE CONCEPT OF CONSTITUTION

Constitution: Character of body as regards health, strength, etc.;
Mental character;
Mode in which State is organized.
Constitutional: Of, inherent in, affecting bodily or mental constitution;
Essential. (Concise Oxford Dictionary)

The concept of 'constitution' is of practical importance not only in homeopathic prescribing, but also in considering the patient's predisposition to illness, its evolution and its natural history in general. Of the brief definitions from the Concise Oxford Dictionary given above, the least obviously appropriate is the one concerning the organization of the State. In fact it provides a helpful analogy if we take it to apply to the whole state of the individual. Our personal constitution is the habitual state of our organism: the organization and interaction of our constituent parts, and the way we are organized to interact with the world. It comprises the basic principles that define us as an individual, just as a political constitution comprises the basic principles that define a State as a political and social institution. In a crisis affecting the State certain of these principles may be reinforced, applied more strictly. Alternatively they may be changed, or the constitution suspended for the duration of the crisis. The constitution may have its weaknesses, flaws and idiosyncrasies. No constitution is perfect. Any constitution may have within it the seeds of potential crisis.

Our individual constitution is very similar. It is the organization of our internal milieu and of our mental and physical responses to our external milieu. These represent our usual equilibrium and include the compensating mechanisms by which we maintain that equilibrium. Our health and personality are more or less stable or precarious according to the state of our constitution, which contains within it the elements of potential crisis or illness. It also includes the resources available to meet external challenge or internal crisis. It has its weaknesses and its strengths.

CONSTITUTION IN HOMEOPATHY

Homeopathy embraces this view of our constitution. It uses it as one perspective within which to view the illness and on which to base a treatment strategy. It also has preventive implications in terms of the vulnerability to illness that it reflects, and the remedial possibilities that constitutional treatment presents.

The constitutional characteristics of the patient prevail in the absence of illness, just as does the usual constitution of the State in the absence of crisis. But they are also aspects of the individual that may intensify when we are ill, so becoming symptoms. Particular physical characteristics, body functions and general reactions, psychological traits and social behaviour that exist as normal traits when we are well may become exaggerated or altered when we are ill. It could be said that one man's constitutional characteristic is another man's symptom. The difference is either a matter of degree or a matter of context. Constitutional characteristics become symptoms if they are exaggerated or diminished in the same individual or if they arise uncharacteristically in someone who usually shows a different tendency. This applies to any symptom that can be a normal trait in some people, but does not, of course, apply to symptoms that exist only as pathological states.

Patterns of constitutional characteristics that are seen consistently and repeatedly in numbers of patients are known as 'constitutional types'. These constitutional patterns have their likeness, their similimum, in the characteristics of homeopathic medicines, just as do clinical pictures. A constitutional pattern of this kind associated with a particular medicine is 'typed' accordingly. Thus we speak of a Pulsatilla type, when we recognize Pulsatilla characteristics in the constitution of a patient, just as we speak of the clinical picture of Pulsatilla when we recognize its characteristic symptoms.

The association between certain constitutional characteristics and particular homeopathic medicines has been made in two ways. The first is the sensitivity shown by certain constitutional types to substances used in experimental pathogenesis (provings). In this case healthy people showing common characteristics have been found to react particularly strongly to test doses of a particular substance. The substance and the medicine derived from it therefore correspond to that constitutional type, and vice versa. In the second case, patients with certain common constitutional characteristics are found to respond particularly well to one specific medicine in the course of treatment. Their common characteristics represent the constitutional type of that medicine. Clinical experience may corroborate the experimental evidence or supplement it with new observations. Alternatively the constitutional type of a medicine may be derived wholly from clinical experience. Thus both the clinical and constitutional pictures of medicines are similarly based on experimental and clinical observations.

RELATIONSHIP BETWEEN CONSTITUTION AND SYMPTOMS

The constitution has already been defined as the state of the individual in the absence of illness. It will reflect traits that make us vulnerable to illness or crisis, but that do not amount to disorder in themselves, or at least are not perceived as disorder. When we become ill the clinical picture may include constitutional features that have become exaggerated. They have become symptoms. A tendency to take offence or to feel self-conscious becomes frankly paranoid; a liking for salt becomes a craving; a warm-blooded person becomes intolerant of any heat; a tendency to burp turns to indigestion; an irregular menstrual cycle becomes extreme; a methodical person becomes obsessional. Alternatively,

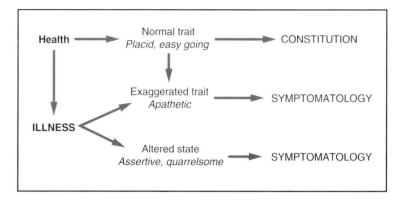

Figure 6.1 Constitution and symptomatology.

the clinical picture may have no relationship to the constitutional picture and become superimposed upon it (Fig. 6.1). For the time being the constitution is suspended, or in more insidious and chronic disorders progressively changed.

A clinical context that demonstrates these alternatives is PMS, particularly the psychological symptoms. When PMS is bad it can seriously disturb a woman's state of mind. She may, for example, become intensely suspicious and jealous, malicious, voluble in her accusation of others and violent. This can be a complete Jekyll and Hyde transformation. On the other hand there can be an underlying constitutional tendency to be rather distrusting, critical, impetuous and talkative. In PMS both possibilities, an exaggeration of existing traits to an intolerable degree or a complete change of temperament, are seen.

DISTINGUISHING BETWEEN THE CLINICAL AND CONSTITUTIONAL PICTURES

There is a degree of confusion in the way that constitutional and clinical characteristics are referred to and used in practice. Some homeopaths, for instance, will describe a prescription based on the totality as a constitutional prescription, whether it corresponds to the constitutional pattern of the individual or not. In addition many homeopaths will include constitutional characteristics in a clinical picture even though they are not a clinical feature of the illness. I believe it is a mistake to do either of these things. The distinction between constitution and symptomatology is useful and should be preserved.

It may often be the case that a patient's constitutional characteristics do fit the pattern of the clinical picture. If so they will, of course, strengthen the similarity of that picture to the medicine that corresponds to it. Nevertheless, it would be better to identify the clinical similimum and the constitutional similimum separately, using the second to corroborate the first, rather than to combine the two as one picture. The danger of combining the two is that the presenting clinical picture and the underlying constitutional pattern may be different. In this case, strong constitutional features may well distort and disguise the true clinical similimum. To use the constitutional perspective to confirm the totality is fine. To include it with the totality is risky.

On the other hand, there are occasions when the clinical picture is vague and inconclusive, and the constitutional picture is vividly clear. If that is *definitely* the case, in other words, if a clinical similimum has been sought conscientiously and not found, then it would be appropriate to prescribe the clearly revealed constitutional similimum.

Does this mean that where clear but different constitutional and clinical pictures coexist then the clinical picture should prevail in the choice of prescription? Where they are seen together at the same time, it should. Where they occur intercurrently because the disorder is episodic and the patient is symptom free in between episodes it may not. The clinical picture at the time of the illness is the immediate expression of the patient's disturbed equilibrium. It reveals the homeopathic stimulus that the patient needs at that time: the medicinal stimulus that faithfully reflects the disorder and disequilibrium on the one hand, and the receptivity and potential for self-regulation on the other. Where that is clearly expressed the clinical similimum is the appropriate response. Where the constitutional similimum corresponds, so much the better – the recovery may be more complete. Where it does not correspond it should be noted for future reference, when the constitutional layer requires attention. If the clinical picture is disregarded and the competing constitutional picture used for the prescription there is a risk of aggravation. The presenting symptoms may be exacerbated but without the subsequent benefits of a true therapeutic aggravation.

TREATING THE VULNERABLE CONSTITUTION

In between different illnesses that occur in the course of our life, or where a particular disorder is episodic (e.g. migraine), there are periods of time with no symptoms and no clinical picture. The constitutional picture that prevails at these times reveals the fundamental vulnerable state of the individual. It reveals the susceptibility to illness rather than its manifestation. In this case the intercurrent and hopefully prophylactic use of the constitutional picture is entirely appropriate. A different similimum may be needed to alleviate the clinical episodes if and when they still occur. One example of an episodic illness in which I have found it consistently effective to treat with the clinical similimum prophylactically in the *absence* of symptoms is PMS. In my own practice I have achieved the best results by prescribing on the clinical picture before ovulation.

IS THERE ALWAYS A CONSTITUTIONAL PICTURE?

Clearly all of us always have a constitution in the general sense in which it has been described. For us to have a constitutional picture in the homeopathic sense, however, our constitutional characteristics must conform to a particular constitutional type – that is, to the similimum of a homeopathic medicine.

There are really two questions here. The first is, do we all have a constitutional type; is a constitutional similimum to be found amongst the repertoire of homeopathic medicines? The second is, do all homeopathic medicines have associated constitutional types? The answer to the first question is 'Perhaps, but it is not always to be found.' The answer to the second is 'Perhaps, but it may not yet have been recognized.'

We often cannot find a medicine that corresponds to the constitutional characteristics of our patient. One reason for this may be that there are no distinctive constitutional characteristics; the patient is, in a sense, too ordinary. This may really be so, or we may have failed to elicit the key characteristics. One way of resolving this is to ask the patient about another member of their family or close circle – 'What is so-and-so like?' 'How is he/she different from you?' This may reveal more distinctive features than the patient has described of themselves. Another way of illuminating the patient's constitution is to ask someone else who knows them well, usually a parent, sibling or spouse. It is surprising, however, how accurate and honest people are in describing themselves and how seldom independent evidence alters the picture. Nevertheless, however we proceed, there are some patients in whom no constitutional characteristics emerge vividly enough to be 'typed'.

The second reason why we may not find a constitutional medicine to correspond to even the most vivid description (accepting the possibility of our simple ignorance) is that one has not been described. That does not mean, however, that it does not exist. There are many 'small medicines' with a limited materia medica and no identifiable constitutional picture, but the suggestion that there are no small medicines, only poorly known ones, has already been mentioned. One of the advances in contemporary homeopathy is the broadening and deepening of our knowledge of small medicines, both by provings and from clinical experience. Constitutional pictures, as well as far richer clinical pictures, are being developed for many of these, and our repertoire of constitutional medicines is consequently being increased.

To restate the question and the answer: Is the constitutional picture of the patient always to be found? No, because it is not always clearly expressed, and because the constitutional potential of many homeopathic medicines is not known.

DOES THE CONSTITUTION CHANGE WITH TIME?

The answer to this question varies according to different views of what our constitution is. The fundamentalist view, so to speak, is that there is one absolutely basic constitution, which is for ever. Other layers may conceal it but it is there if we can find it. This is an esoteric view, sometimes with metaphysical overtones. The view that satisfies the practical experience of the majority, and indeed common sense, is that the constitution does change in some people, while it remains the same in others. Certain predictable sequences of change occurring as a child matures towards adult life have been described in terms of their corresponding homeopathic medicines. Circumstances, environment and experience may fundamentally change an individual's constitution over the years, as, surely, may the healing process itself.

In any case, this is a largely unhelpful speculation if the aim of homeopathy is to reflect faithfully in our treatment the picture that confronts us at the time.

CONSTITUTIONAL AND CLINICAL CARICATURES

There is a temptation to turn the identification of constitutional types and their related clinical picture into a sort of party game by creating caricatures. Teachers of homeopathy often lead us into this habit, because it is fun, it makes a useful point, and because like all caricatures they are based on accurate observation. Margaret Tyler's description of Sepia is one of the most notorious examples of this practice. Beginning, 'Sepia has been called the Washer woman's Remedy. Picture her . . . the sallow, tired mother of a big family on washing day', it continues for a page and a half of vivid prose 'the worry of the children is more than she can bear. . . . Oh, how she wants to run away and leave it all. . . . Her husband comes in; she has no smile to greet his. . . . He looks at her sadly. Her dull face has lost its contour, its bloom, its pleasing lines.' (Tyler M 1952).

Descriptions like this convey parts of the picture, pieces of the jigsaw, unforgettably. The trouble is that they are so vivid that they can blind us to other possibilities when we look at real patients. We may wrongly exclude Sepia from consideration when we do not see them, or equally wrongly base a prescription of Sepia on a few features of the caricature that could belong to quite a different picture. These caricatures are a mixed blessing. They can open our eyes to a particular picture, and even make possible some dramatic 'spot diagnoses'. But they can be seriously distracting. A colleague has a lecture slide that makes this point charmingly. It shows a patient who has responded extremely well to Pulsatilla, which is caricatured as a fair-haired, blue-eyed girl. The slide shows a delightful West Indian child with, of course, the blackest hair and brownest eyes you can imagine.

MORPHOLOGICAL TYPES

One view of the constitution has been based exclusively on the physique of the individual. These morphological types associate certain medicines with certain patterns of anatomical structure. The longilinear or Phosphoric constitution is described by

Jouanny (1980): 'Above normal height with development in the vertical direction. The weight is less than appropriate for the height, making the patient look thin, and perhaps hunched. The face is triangular and long (dolicocephalic). . . . The hands are long and elegant. . . . There is relative hypo-laxity of the ligaments.' He contrasts this with other types such as the Carbonic constitution: 'Height less than average . . . face square or round'. He also describes the pathological tendencies and neuropsychic behaviour (psychological traits) of each type.

The morphological approach is not much used in British homeopathy. It does, however, offer another perspective, which may guide us towards the right prescription, but like constitutional caricatures can be misleading.

CONSTITUTION AND TERRAIN

The concept of 'terrain' is applied more commonly in France than in Britain. It is closely similar to constitution but places greater emphasis on the factors that predispose to illness. As the word implies it describes the landscape, and both landscape and the political definition of constitution used above are helpful metaphors. Both describe our day to day functional state in the absence of particular illness. Both describe our fundamental susceptibility to illness. Where constitution tends towards portraiture, or the more literary style of Margaret Tyler, terrain tends towards the more clinical view of health status. It relates more to the nutritional and ecological predisposing factors that are involved in the aetiology, causing an unhealthy or weakened terrain.

THE CONSTITUTION IN CHRONIC ILLNESS

Inevitably many chronic illnesses eventually erode and change the habitual constitutional state of the individual that prevailed before the illness developed. That earlier state of the patient and the manifestations of the illness may have become indistinguishably intermingled on every level. In these circumstances it is not realistic to make a distinction between the clinical and constitutional pictures.

The key points regarding constitution are summarized in Box 6.1.

Box 6.1 Constitution

- The constitution is the habitual state of the patient.
- Constitutional characteristics may be reflected in the symptomatology if they become exaggerated in the course of the illness.
- Prescriptions may be based on the constitutional similimum when it corresponds to the clinical similimum, or in the absence of a clinical similimum because the patient is symptom free or the clinical picture is indistinct.
- A constitutional prescription should not be made if it conflicts with the current clinical picture.
- It is not always possible to identify the constitutional picture of an individual.
- Constitutional characteristics may become subsumed in the clinical picture of chronic illness.

THE CONVENTIONAL VIEW OF CONSTITUTION

Personality, lifestyle, including diet, genetic and congenital factors and environmental influences are important in all conventional medicine for a proper understanding of diagnosis and aetiology, for prognosis and for planning treatment and preventive care. These are all aspects of constitution, but the concept as an integrated whole is not used. Thomas Sydenham, who has been mentioned earlier (Ch. 1), recognized the existence of the 'epidemic constitution', a common susceptibility to disease within groups of the population. In fact he reintroduced this concept from the teachings of Hippocrates, and such was his stature that he was known as the English Hippocrates. Hippocrates, the 'father of medicine', was the first physician to promote the principle of treating like with like. It is challenging to speculate what epidemiological insights and preventive possibilities might be gained by a systematic investigation of the significance of constitution in the homeopathic sense in the evolution of illness.

REFERENCES

Jouanny J 1980 The essential of homeopathic therapeutics. Boiron, Bordeaux
Tyler M 1952 Homeopathic drug pictures, 3rd edn. Health Science Press, Holsworthy, pp 738–739

FURTHER READING

Foubister D 1969 Constitutional types: an evaluation of this concept in relation to homeopathic prescribing. British Homeopathic Journal 58: 77–81

7

Aetiology

The view of health and illness presented so far is of continuing evolution. It implies that none of us is ever in perfect health. Even when we regard ourselves as well we possess inherent traits or constitutional susceptibilities that make us vulnerable to illness. This state of affairs is continuously changing, for better or worse, depending on the healing or pathogenic influence of circumstances and life events. The process leads to occasional, or if we are unfortunate frequent or persistent, states of illness or disorder. All these episodes are seen in homeopathy as facets of a coherent underlying state of disorder. No symptom or disorder arises independently of the whole.

The aetiological factors that influence this process are no different from those that we would recognize in conventional medicine – familial and congenital, infectious, toxic and traumatic, environmental, social, psychological, spiritual. Some of these will be predisposing factors, determining the soil in which the illness may develop. Some will be provoking or precipitating factors, the seed from which the particular illness will develop at a particular time or over the course of time.

NEVER WELL SINCE

There are many instances of long-term morbidity arising from aetiological factors that are no longer active. The syndrome 'never well since' is well recognized. It may follow any illness or event that significantly disturbs us physiologically or psychologically, any sufficient constitutional disturbance. It may consist of any permutation of psychological or somatic features. Where the causative agent is still present and active we try to remove it. The only area of long-term morbidity of this kind commonly subject to intervention that is directly related to an aetiology that is no longer active is psychological. Chronic psychological and psychosomatic illness may be addressed by counselling or psychotherapy, which explores the formative psychological experience and seeks to heal its adverse long-term effects. Physical treatments for such psychosomatic sequelae, including psychotropic medication, do not of course address the cause. Nor does conventional treatment of the somatic consequences of physical aetiology that is itself no longer active. It can only seek to remedy what has happened, not to reverse the process by which it happened.

Conventional medicine is sometimes ambivalent towards somatic 'never well since' syndromes. Unless it is possible to demonstrate actual physiological disturbance directly attributable to the causal event, the problem is likely to be diagnosed as psychoneurotic. An example from the past was chronic brucellosis. The 16th edition of Conybeare's textbook of medicine, published in 1975, reads, 'Chronic Brucellosis may simulate psycho-neurotic illness. It is important to realize that psycho-neurosis may mistakenly be attributed to brucella infection long "burnt out", and conversely that a diagnosis of neurotic illness may be made when the true cause of the symptoms is chronic brucellosis' (Jamieson 1975). We have learned this lesson, but it is likely that this applies to many instances of 'never well since X', when X is mistakenly believed to be burnt out. It may indeed be burnt out in the sense that its active features are no longer to be detected, as when the serology returns to normal in brucellosis. But this is a very different matter from assuming that the subtle physiological consequences of the event are eradicated.

In this case we are talking about the direct physiological consequences in the mind or body of physical factors. The other face of the coin concerns the role of psychological factors in the aetiology of chronic physical illness. We may suspect it in the evolution of rheumatoid arthritis, multiple sclerosis, cancer or any chronic disease or dysfunction in particular patients. The role may be major or minor. We might see it as precipitating or predisposing, interacting with pre-existing conditions or subsequent events to set up the specific disease process. If such an aetiology is clearly perceived we might try to address it directly by psychological means. The chances are, however, that a causative factor of this kind will not be sought or addressed. Few physicians dealing with chronic illnesses have the opportunity to explore their psychological components, even if they do have the inclination. As our understanding of the interaction of psychological, neuropeptide and immunological mechanisms increases there may be greater motivation to include psychological factors in the management of these illnesses. How to do so would be the big question.

Many doctors would consider the circumstances attending the evolution of a long-term illness as aetiological only if there is a demonstrable and direct pathogenic association with it. Many doctors also find the distinction and interrelation of psyche and soma difficult to interpret and to manage. Homeopathy does not accept any such dichotomy because it regards the two as intimately and inextricably related facets of the whole in every case. It regards all illness in that sense as psychosomatic. Similarly it regards all the attendant circumstances in the evolution of an illness as significant if their impact upon the patient on any level has been significant. Where this clear association is found, homeopathy is often able to respond directly to the aetiological factor with the appropriately indicated medicine (Fig. 7.1). The treatment reflects the cause, however distant the event, however long since the active aetiological process ceased.

AETIOLOGICAL PRESCRIBING

Whatever our medical discipline, conventional or complementary, understanding of constitutional and aetiological factors related to personality, lifestyle, diet, environment, etc. allows us to make appropriate interventions through education and counselling. These may be therapeutic or preventive, and focused on the individual or the community. Constitutional and aetiological 'prescriptions' of this kind are a familiar part of medical practice.

The difference in the homeopathic approach is twofold. First, it includes the perception of constitutional characteristics as an

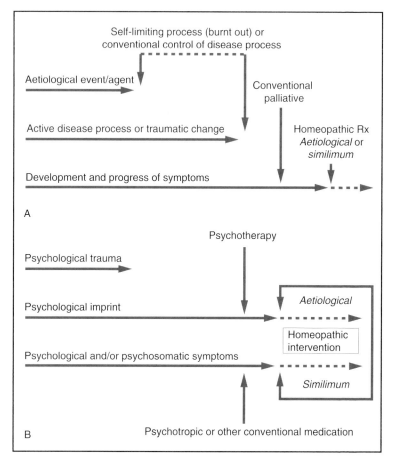

Figure 7.1 The role of aetiological prescribing in homeopathy. A: Role in physical illness. B: Role in psychological illness.

integrated whole and of aetiological factors as a cumulative influence on a person's health history. Secondly, constitutional patterns and aetiological factors are used as indications for specific homeopathic prescriptions.

A recurrent theme of this book is the *fact* of the phenomena to be observed in the patient in the course and manifestation of the illness and in response to the homeopathic intervention. The existence of these phenomena does not depend on the role of the specific or non-specific elements of the intervention. We do not have to be able to prove their attribution in order to recognize that they occur. They are valid and valuable as clinical observations in their own right.

When we base a homeopathic intervention on the aetiology of the illness and the patient recovers, the recovery is a reality irrespective of the relationship of the actual role of the medicine in relation to the aetiological event. Whether it is a placebo response, or a psychotherapeutic response, or a response to an active medicine specifically indicated by the aetiology, we have equal reason to be pleased and the process of recovery that we observe is equally valid in itself. One way or another we have stimulated a change by exploiting the aetiological insight. In aetiological prescribing, however, the full significance of the changes we observe cannot be realized unless we are certain of the specific efficacy of the medicine in relation to the aetiological factor. (This is also true of other prescribing strategies, as will be discussed later.)

The recovery of patients from chronic disorders following a homeopathic prescription based on aetiological indications is common. To demonstrate beyond doubt that this process is achieved by directly antidoting, so to speak, the particular aetiological influence, even though it is no longer active, would be of profound significance, not only for the reputation of homeopathy but for our whole understanding of disease processes. Homeopathic interventions based on the aetiological rationale described in the following pages are certainly effective. Their implications deserve serious consideration whatever the mechanisms involved. The possibility that the action of the specific aetiological medicine constitutes one mechanism is of the greatest importance and requires the fullest investigation.

HISTORICAL PATTERNS
Family history

It is unusual for a patient to volunteer a family history of syphilis. From a homeopathic point of view such a history is believed to be of particular importance because it accounts for one of the powerful traits, or miasms, that predispose to illness in later generations even when there is no congenital infection. Early in my career a young woman with chronic urticaria who had read books on homeopathy spontaneously reported her family history of syphilis. Working in general practice I did not have time for a lengthy consultation and was glad of such a vivid aetiological clue. The appropriate nosode (medicine derived from diseased tissue or products of disease) was prescribed (Syphilinum) and the urticaria resolved. It is tempting to say that Syphilinum effected a complete cure. But of course there are psychodynamic reasons why the symbolic administration of the antidote to the disease of which the patient was obviously very conscious might have effected a powerful placebo response.

Nevertheless, a strong family history suggesting a trait such as this is a clear indication of the need for the specific nosode at some point in the treatment strategy (Fig. 7.2). If the trait is deep seated the treatment may not be complete without it. The disease processes underlying these major traits all have their associated nosodes. Those most commonly used on the basis of the family history are probably the Tuberculinum group, derived from tuberculous material. The incidence of this family history is high. Most full-time homeopaths probably encounter it at least once a week. A multicentre placebo-controlled trial of the use of Tuberculinum in appropriate patients would be feasible and of great interest. The clinical results of its use in a wide variety of morbidity are certainly striking.

The presence of a single disease trait strongly represented in the family is one kind of familial aetiology. 'Strongly represented' means present in a number of family members or across a

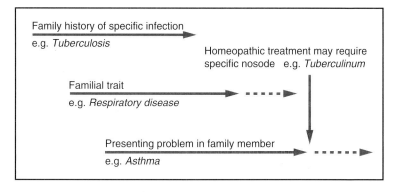

Figure 7.2   Aetiological treatment relating to family history.

number of generations, or close exposure of the patient to a carrier without transmission of the disease. Another aetiological pattern is the coexistence of certain different diseases within the family history. One example is the coexistence of some permutation of carcinoma, diabetes, pernicious anaemia, thyroid disease or tuberculosis, within or across generations. This pattern is an indication for a prescription of Carcinosin (derived from carcinomatous material).

Personal history and diathesis

Specific diseases occurring in the personal history may have similar significance even when they have not precipitated the 'never well since' scenario. A healed focus in the lung may be an incidental finding on chest X-ray. This might be an indication for Tuberculinum, as also might be history of a positive Mantoux or Heaf test, particularly if the clinical picture shows the relevant pattern or diathesis.

The concept of diathesis is related to the familial traits described above and to the concepts of constitution and terrain. 'Constitutional predisposition to disease, etc.' is the Concise Oxford Dictionary definition. Diathesis is used most often in homeopathy to refer to the evidence of this predisposition in the health history and/or current health of the individual rather than in the family. A pattern of illness may be said to reflect a particular diathesis, the underlying predisposition to that illness.

The tubercular diathesis is one such pattern. Its clinical features are similar to those that might be seen in a tubercular patient, such as night sweats, recurrent or chronic respiratory disorder, lymphadenopathy. Migraine is also considered to be part of this diathesis. Where this pattern is seen in a patient Tuberculinum may be a necessary part of the regime.

The various books of classical materia medica use the word diathesis very freely to describe the pattern of illness in a patient, either the clinical picture at one time or the history as a whole. They speak of the haemorrhagic diathesis, the uric acid diathesis, the rheumatic diathesis, as well as the tubercular diathesis and the sycotic diathesis. This usage often seems to have a purely descriptive function, rather than any aetiological significance. The therapeutic value of the concept, however, lies in the evidence that the diathesis provides of the predisposition to a particular pattern of illness, its association with a particular disease process, and the opportunity to reflect this in the choice of medicine.

A diathesis might, of course, also be seen in the pattern of illness in the family history. The tubercular trait may be revealed in the prevalence of the relevant symptomatology or types of morbidity in the family background when there is no known history of tuberculosis. The familial trait may be seen in the absence of the individual diathesis, or vice versa, or both may be seen together in the family and personal history of one individual. Both would be attributed to the influences of the same 'miasm'.

Miasms

Miasms are the traditional homeopathic classification of fundamental disease processes. They are the expression of morbific (pathogenic) influences affecting populations, families or individuals. Traditionally they have been associated with particular diseases on the basis of a direct aetiological link. Thus the syphilitic miasm was seen as directly attributable to the prevalence of syphilis in the population at the end of the 18th century when Hahnemann was investigating and developing the principles of homeopathy. His interpretation of his observations was obviously influenced by the culture and state of medical science of his day. The aetiological associations that he proposed are not taken literally today, but the existence of certain coherent classes of disease process is. Patterns of disease whose pathology and symptomatology show common characteristics, behaviour and evolution can be distinguished in patients and are reflected in the materia medica. This is not a nosology based on present day concepts of pathology so much as on clinical observation, but pathology is certainly part of the picture. Proliferative and exudative pathologies belong to the sycotic pattern for example, and destructive and degenerative pathologies to the syphilitic.

The value of the miasmatic principle, therefore, is its classification of disease behaviour and of the homeopathic medicines, which correspond to particular patterns of disease behaviour. These patterns can be seen running through the history of individuals and their families, and of populations subject to common pathogenic influences. They have an aetiological role as well as being reflected in the current or recurrent clinical picture. The recognition of these patterns permits the choice of a homeopathic medicine associated with them. This pattern of illness or disease behaviour may be sufficient indication for a particular medicine in its own right, or may be a pointer towards one of the medicines suggested by the presenting clinical picture.

ONSET

Circumstances surrounding the onset of illness are of importance to our understanding and management of it, whatever the clinical context of our work. We always need to know why this patient became ill in this way at this time. Why was it this patient and not another who may have been exposed to the same circumstances, the same endemic or epidemic influence? Why did it occur in this way, with this symptomatology or disorder and not with some other clinical picture? Why does A develop one syndrome and B another in response to similar circumstances (stress, bereavement, infection, etc.)? Why did the condition to which the patient is obviously predisposed become manifest now, rather than last year or next year? Why did this patient with familial diabetes exhibit it in her thirties, and that one in his teens?

The extent to which we explore these circumstances, however, and the emphasis we put upon them vary considerably. Where one aetiological factor is obvious we may disregard the possible influence of others. Where the familial aetiology of diabetes is obvious we may not consider the question 'Why *now*? ' to be relevant. Where the pathology is commonplace or not very serious we may not feel we need to ask 'Why' at all. Above all perhaps, when we believe we can do nothing useful with the information we have no reason to elicit it. Identifying a specific infection that may have precipitated the onset of frank diabetes is essential if we are to control it. Where no such specific and remediable factors are implicated we may not be prompted to undertake the lateral thinking.

In homeopathy these questions 'Why?' surrounding the onset of a particular illness or the start of a sequence of illnesses in a previously more healthy person are critically important. They need to be asked whatever the pathology and whatever other aetiological factors are known to be operating (Fig. 7.3). The most immediately practical reason is that the essential prescription may need to be based upon them. The 'never well since' scenario has been discussed already, and will often be reported spontaneously because the impact of the event and the subsequent change are usually clear in the patient's mind. Often, however, the significance of events may not be so apparent. Clinicians should be aware of the importance of transitional events in people's lives (going to school, leaving home, starting work, marriage, parenthood, retirement, etc.) and their possible aetiological effects. Patients may not be. They may take them for granted and make no association with subsequent changes in well-being. Any episode of illness, any life event, any psychological process, any change in our internal or external milieu may precipitate change in our health. Their impact and the reasons for it may be elicited only by careful enquiry. We need to ask, 'Was there anything else going on in your life when this (the illness) started?' 'Could anything else in your life have upset the apple cart, lowered your resistance, destabilized you?' The choice of words will need to be tailored to the individual.

We may need to pinpoint the beginning of the illness more clearly with questions such as, 'When did you last feel really well?' We may then find that the presenting problem arose from a background of undifferentiated poor health. The patient may

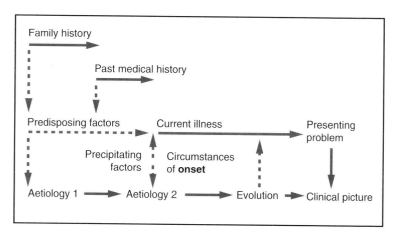

Figure 7.3   The circumstances of the onset of illness are an important part of the aetiological pattern.

not relate this to their current problem, but this was perhaps the beginning of it and the key aetiological factor may lie there. Having identified the starting point of the illness and the events associated with it we then need to understand the impact of those events. What were their physical and psychological repercussions? Any significant event may have either or both, probably both.

INFECTION

Knowledge of an infectious cause for an illness is of value homeopathically in two ways. The 'never well since' syndrome arising from infection has already been described. This is a syndrome in which the precipitating infectious agent is no longer active. Any infection may have had a precipitating role of this kind from commonplace childhood infections such as measles, through gonorrhoea and glandular fever to toxoplasmosis and tuberculosis. In any of these cases the use of an appropriate nosode may be essential to full recovery, even if the clinical similimum produces some improvement.

In active infections, particularly if recurrent, a homeopathic preparation of the infecting organism (the nosode) may be a valuable adjunct to the clinical similimum. This is, of course, technically isopathy not homeopathy: the use of the substance that is the same as the causative agent, rather than one producing a similar clinical effect. Examples are preparations of *Herpes simplex* in cold sores, *Candida* in thrush, *Staphylococcus* in infected eczema and *Escherichia coli*, *Pseudomonas* or other organisms in the recurrent infections of neurogenic bladder.

IMMUNIZATION

A corollary of the use of homeopathy in conditions of infectious aetiology is the question of its prophylactic use. It is believed that preparations of the appropriate organism may be an effective alternative for routine immunization. There has been considerable popular interest in this possibility because of anxieties about the adverse effects of conventional immunization. Many non-medically qualified homeopaths and some doctors believe that routine immunization has long-term deleterious effects on the immune system; that, while it is effective in providing specific immunity, it predisposes to a variety of illnesses that involve some disorder of the immune system later in life. The great majority of homeopathic doctors either do not accept this argument, or consider that what evidence does point in this direction is insufficient to outweigh the obvious benefits of immunization.

The effectiveness of 'homeopathic immunization' is doubtful. Attempts to investigate it in whooping cough have been inconclusive because of problems with numbers of subjects and diagnosis of the condition (English 1987, 1992). Clinical experience is particularly unreliable in this situation. Nevertheless, many of us do use prophylactic regimes where conventional immunization is actually contraindicated or refused by the parents. Accurate homeopathic prescribing for the condition itself if it does arise is likely to be more effective.

ALLERGY

Isopathy is commonly used in the treatment of allergies. Glasgow Homeopathic Hospital has extensive experience of desensitization with homeopathic preparations of allergens (Kayne and Beattie 1996). The three placebo-controlled studies published by David Reilly, two of them in the Lancet, and conducted in Glasgow used isopathic preparations in allergic states (Reilly and Taylor 1985, Reilly et al 1986, 1994). All three refuted the hypothesis that ultramolecular homeopathic dilutions are no more effective than placebo. The alternative conclusion is that the double-blind placebo-controlled trial is not, after all, a reliable test of efficacy (Editorial Lancet 1994)!

An allergy is evidence of an unstable immune system. Its treatment may require a comprehensive strategy of homeopathic treatment that takes account of the full clinical picture and any other perspectives and aetiological factors that are relevant. Sometimes the appropriate 'local' prescription or the use of the isopathic preparation of the allergen is effective on its own. Some allergic or hypersensitivity states are precipitated by other specific illnesses or psychological factors. The patient mentioned in Chapter 3 who took 3 hours to give a history is an example. Psychological trauma in pregnancy was a distant cause of her hypersensitivities, and homeopathic desensitization would not have resolved them. As part of a treatment strategy, however, homeopathic allergens can be very effective. And where the allergy is an isolated clinical phenomenon in a patient who at that time is otherwise well, they can be effectively used alone. Specific reactions to domestic animals and horses, milk, sugar, dust, feathers and plants of various kinds (to name but a few) are commonly treated in this way. Homeopathic preparations of pollens are made from the same source material as were conventional desensitizing preparations in the days before their dangers led to their withdrawal from use.

IATROGENIC REACTIONS

The treatment of adverse reactions to conventional drugs with their isopathic counterparts has been practised increasingly in the past 15 years. It has also been used to assist withdrawal of benzodiazepine tranquillizers. I have rarely used the method except palliatively in cancer patients receiving radiotherapy and chemotherapy, where I am impressed by the benefits of Radium Bromide and Phosphorus respectively in reducing the adverse effects of treatment.

PHYSICAL TRAUMA

The staff and district midwives looking after patients at our cottage hospital gave great encouragement to my early use of homeopathy in general practice. Arnica tablets were kept there for relief of perineal trauma after delivery in my own patients and I was surprised one day to find the stock severely depleted. It turned out that the other midwives had been helping themselves for the benefit of their patients, so impressed were they by its efficacy.

The value of Arnica in all trauma, especially soft tissue damage, is widely known and accepted – and extremely easily tested in the common traumas of everyday life and sport. Any sceptic could mount their own double-blind trial within their own family or rugby club if they felt so inclined. The effects of Arnica are so convincing that I would consider myself negligent not to recommend it to a patient preoperatively. Its prophylactic and therapeutic use in assisting the control of pain and recovery after surgery is a consistently good source of anecdotal evidence.

There are a number of homeopathic medicines indicated for

specific types of trauma (Box 7.1). Several, like Arnica, can be used prophylactically. One of particular interest is Staphysagria. It is indicated for injuries that are particularly intrusive, that to some extent violate the person. These include surgical incisions, cystoscopy and urethal dilatation and sexual abuse and rape. It is also indicated for honeymoon cystitis. 'Never well since' any episode of physical trauma may respond to Arnica. The traumatic event may be distant in time. Surprising results may be obtained in the treatment of the long-term sequelae of head injuries with Arnica or Natrum sulphuricum, for example.

Box 7.1   Homeopathic medicines associated with trauma

Natrum sulphuricum	Head injury
Aconite	Eye injury
Ledum	Penetrating injury, bites and stings
Staphysagria	Incised wounds, urethral dilatation
Rhus toxicodendron	Strains and sprains
Calendula	Abrasions
Hypericum	Injury to nerves, to coccyx
Symphytum	Fractures

PSYCHOLOGICAL TRAUMA AND DEPRIVATION

Box 7.2 shows a selection of psychological factors listed in the homeopathic literature that are known indications for particular medicines. They encompass most kinds of psychological trauma and stress, including experiences of loss and emotional deprivation. There are numerous medicines associated with these. They are extremely valuable in homeopathy and are frequently indicated because psychological distress has such a high incidence and prevalent aetiological role in our culture.

Box 7.2   Psychological stresses indicating particular homeopathic medicines

'Ailments from . . .'
Anger, suppressed anger, indignation
Disappointment, embarrassment, grief
Homesickness, disappointed love
Anxiety, fear, bad news
Rudeness, scorn, mortification

Their effective use requires the same insight and understanding of psychological nuance as would be required in counselling or psychotherapy. And of course the process of eliciting their indications is a psychotherapeutic process in itself. This would seem to make it particularly difficult to disentangle any specific effect of the medicine from the psychological effect of the intervention. Interestingly this is not necessarily the case. Those of us who have experience of using psychotherapy with and without homeopathy are quite clear about the difference homeopathy makes. In both instances we are giving time, attention and (we hope) empathy. We are exploring the psychodynamics similarly in both cases. In both cases we may be giving a pill, psychotropic or homeopathic. Irrespective of their specific effects the placebo power of psychotropic drugs is known, even down to the best choice of colour for antidepressant and tranquillizer tablets (Anton et al 1996). The appearance of homeopathic tablets is considerably less impressive! These similarities emphasize the additional benefits of the homeopathic prescription. In the case of psychosomatic symptoms considerable insight, reconciliation and healing can be achieved on the psychological level without relief of the physical symptoms. Homeopathy can be particularly helpful in this context.

As these remarks imply, to choose the correct homeopathic medicine we must understand the dynamics well. The reference in Chapter 4 (Language and meaning, p. 59) to the fear of crowds is an example of this. Consider also the effect on a woman of moving house. Women frequently have much more emotional investment in their homes and their locality than men, and when there has been any depth of attachment moving away from these roots can be a real grief. On the other hand, if the move was precipitated by a change in her husband's occupation she may be angry and resentful, with him or his firm, or whoever is responsible. She herself may not at first recognize these reactions in herself, let alone as a cause of her illness. Sensitivity and imagination, and a knowledge of the possibilities, are necessary to help her towards the correct interpretation. There is not an entry in the literature for 'ailments from moving house'. If there was it would need breaking down into its component emotions, or would need to include the set of medicines that cover the possible reactions. There is not an entry for ailments from resentment either, which is a notable and strange omission from the repertory language. It can be remedied by reference to entries for anger and indignation and such like alternatives. On the other hand there is an entry for 'ailments from disappointed love'. An analysis of the different nuances of this experience represented in the different medicines associated with it can occupy a 2-hour seminar with no difficulty.

Arnica, the famous medicine for physical trauma, is also indicated for psychological trauma. If a patient complains of feeling emotionally battered, they may well need Arnica. Staphysagria is also found in this category of medicines and is frequently indicated. Here the psychological trauma involves wounded feelings, an element of humiliation, an insult to a person's sense of worth; it is usually associated with suppressed anger because of it. A patient with acne rosacea failed to respond to a number of well-indicated medicines until the degree of humiliation involved in her partner's treatment of her and its relationship to the onset of her rosacea became apparent. The Staphysagria was dramatically effective. Or was it the psychotherapeutic and placebo content of the consultation that revealed the indications for it? The question is important. Certainly when the condition began to recur Staphysagria was again effective, and no further discussion of emotional themes took place. The ability to discriminate confidently between the effects of different aspects of the intervention may not improve the outcome, but is essential to our understanding of the role of the prescription.

When there has been an appreciable psychotherapeutic content to a consultation it may be better not to prescribe homeopathically. Partly this is because it is better not to give further stimulus to a process that already has some momentum; partly it is because the separate influence of the two activities could not be distinguished in the outcome. This was the case with a patient whose guttate psoriasis turned out to be associated with sexual guilt. One long consultation revealed and resolved this, and the psoriasis itself resolved in a few days, with no prescription. Guttate psoriasis is a more labile condition than rosacea, and the mechanism of recovery in the two cases could have been the same or different.

Here again we are faced with uncertainty. Is change effected by placebo, by psychotherapy, by the homeopathic medicine or by all of them? And once again the point is that change *is* effected, and more effectively than in other clinical settings. We need to study the implications. We need to know why.

The above examples of aetiological events indicating homeopathic medicines are by no means exhaustive. Such events are important in the homeopathic interpretation of the case, and aetiological prescribing is of great value. But again it needs to be pointed out that such events are only part of the story. The same aetiological event will not affect everybody, and those whom it does affect will be affected in different ways. It is one thread in the tapestry of the whole clinical picture. When we prescribe on an aetiological indication we are not, therefore, simply antidoting a particular event, except in the case of a circumscribed isopathic indication. We are also treating the susceptibility to that event (Fig. 7.4). The medicine indicated may reflect the whole clinical or constitutional picture, encompassing both the susceptibility to the illness and the manifestation of it, and the event, the soil and the seed. Or it may be dealing only with one level or layer of illness. The aetiological dimension must therefore be kept in perspective.

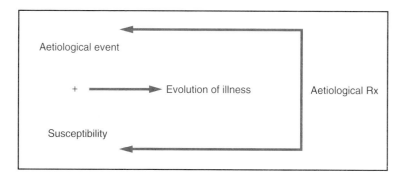

Figure 7.4 Aetiological prescriptions treat the susceptibility as well as the process.

REFERENCES

Anton J, Roos P, de Vries A, Kleijnen J 1996 Effect of colour of drugs: systematic review of perceived effect of drugs and their effectiveness. British Medical Journal 313: 1624–1626
Editorial 1994 Reilly's challenge. Lancet 344: 1585

English J 1987 Pertussin 30—preventive for whooping cough? A pilot study. British Homeopathic Journal 76: 61–65

English J 1992 The issue of immunisation. British Homeopathic Journal 81: 161–163

Jamieson W 1975 Diseases due to infection. In: Mann W (ed) Conybeare's textbook of medicine, 16th edn. Churchill Livingstone, New York, p 57

Kayne S, Beattie N 1996 Preliminary results from an investigation of three different isopathic dose regimes used in the treatment of allergy. Communications; British Homeopathy Research Group 24: 26–29

Reilly D, Taylor M 1985 Potent placebo or potency? A proposed study model with initial findings using homeopathically prepared pollens in hay fever. British Homeopathic Journal 74: 65–75

Reilly D, Taylor M, McSharry C, Aitchison T 1986 Is homeopathy a placebo response? Controlled trial of homeopathic potency, with pollen in hay fever as model. Lancet 1986 ii: 881–886

Reilly D, Taylor M, Beattie N et al 1994 Is evidence for homeopathy reproducible? Lancet 334: 1600–1606

FURTHER READING

Brostoff J 1986 Low dose desensitisation. Communications of the British Homeopathy Research Group 16: 21–24

Foubister D 1963 Past history in homeopathic prescribing. British Homeopathic Journal 52: 81–91

8

When to use homeopathy?

The next chapter provides an overview of treatment strategies in homeopathy, but for many users the most basic strategic issue is whether and when to use it in the first place. It concerns all those who use homeopathy occasionally rather than routinely. This includes general practice homeopaths, any doctor considering referral for homeopathy and, of course, patients themselves. They will need to understand the possible role of homeopathy in different clinical situations and who has the experience to manage the problem.

CLINICAL SETTING AND LEVELS OF EXPERTISE

It is important to get the use of homeopathy in perspective. It is used in first aid and self-help situations by people who buy the medicines over the counter (OTC). It is used by chiropodists, dentists, nurses and vets. Amongst medically qualified practitioners it is used predominately in general practice. It is used by doctors who have specialized in its study and work as consultants in the health service and in private practice. And it is used by non-medically qualified professional (NMQP) homeopaths. These usually work privately and independently of the health service, but a few are now integrated within NHS primary care. Each context requires its particular repertoire of knowledge and expertise, and it is essential that the use of homeopathy does not exceed the relevant bounds of competence of the user or the setting. This is obviously true of the practice of any medical skill. Anyone may remove a splinter from a finger, but most of us are ill advised to attempt to remove a foreign body from the cornea.

There is a tendency to elitism among some practitioners of homeopathy who regard its in-depth study as the only proper course and its off-the-cuff use in general practice as a travesty. This is a grave mistake. The constraints of time can be a real limiting factor, but appropriate training can make a widely useful repertoire available to the GP and can make the GP a very useful homeopath within those constraints. Excellent programmes with this objective are being developed in the UK and Europe (Reilly & Taylor 1993, Smulders M 1996 awaiting publication). Experience can extend and deepen this repertoire to such an extent that GPs become able to make interventions in a wide range of morbidity, both acute and chronic. In a study performed in the UK in 1987, two of the 49 participating GPs used homeopathy in at least 80% of their routine consultations. The average was 25% (Swayne 1989, 1990).

Protocols are being developed to make homeopathy a convenient response to the basic health care needs of developing countries. The role of homeopathy in this context has been investigated in the treatment of malaria (Erp & Brands 1996) and acute childhood diarrhoea (Jacobs, Jimenez & Gloyd 1993, Jacobs et al 1994, Jacobs, Jimenez & Malthouse 1997 awaiting publication). The cholera epidemic in Peru in 1991 provided an opportunity for homeopathy to support the other health care initiatives (Gaucher et al 1993). It was of course cholera and other devastating epidemic conditions that were the occasion of some of homeopathy's most striking early achievements.

The OTC sale of homeopathic medicines is a rapidly growing market in the UK. We do not know how appropriate or effective is the use of these, but their popularity implies that they achieve at least some benefit. The disadvantage of this trend is that the availability of these medicines can lead people to underestimate the complexity of the choice of the correct prescription.

The scope for the use of homeopathy is then, very wide. Although its regular use in the treatment of chronic illness does require specialist expertise and usually time, appropriate training and criteria can make it very useful on every level of medical intervention. The comments that follow should be read with that perspective in mind.

POTENTIAL

Homeopathy appears to act by mobilizing, or enhancing, natural processes of healing, regeneration, integration, or compensation. There are very few disorders where one or more of these processes cannot achieve an improvement in the clinical state of the patient. Hence there are very few clinical situations in which homeopathy does not have some role. But its role will not be widely accepted in the vast range of morbidity where it could be but rarely is used in the UK, until three things happen. Homeopaths must develop sufficient expertise in the clinical situations they seldom see, particularly acute ones. These will include acute illnesses that frequently occur for which a conventional remedy is readily, and perhaps inappropriately, available. Other clinicians must gain experience of the effects of homeopathy in a wide range of morbidity giving homeopaths the opportunity to collaborate with them in these areas. And formal research is needed to support that clinical experience.

Formal research is not the be-all and end-all, certainly not double-blind trials. The influence of clinical experience has already been mentioned (Ch. 1, p. 6), and more might be achieved to establish the value of homeopathy by clinical collaboration and audit rather than formal trials. But both controlled trials and well-planned observational research are still essential. They require opportunity (including goodwill), expertise and money, and the combination of the three has been scarce in the history of homeopathy. The cultural change that is taking place with regard to the legitimacy of complementary medicine should help. Compare the tone of the two BMA reports on the subject, separated by an interval of 7 years (British Medical Association 1986, 1993).

LIMITATIONS

The few clinical situations in which homeopathy probably does not have a role include failure of major endocrine systems, certainly in the early stages of treatment. This does mean failure rather than early dysfunction, which can be helped. But where the pituitary, thyroid, adrenal, or islet cells are already substantially impaired homeopathy may have no role until body tissues are responding to replacement of the missing hormone. Sexual hormone imbalance and menopausal syndrome do, however, benefit from homeopathy. Deficiencies of essential nutrients (vitamins, minerals, etc.) similarly disqualify homeopathy from an active role until they are replaced, unless the deficiency is due to inefficient uptake of an essential ingredient that is present in the diet where absorption may be improved. Homeopathy may help symptomatically and may enhance the rate of recovery from these major endocrine and deficiency disorders, but it is best regarded as second phase treatment. Another area where homeopathy may not have a role is in specific degenerative disorders where tissue healing is not a possibility and there are no compensatory mechanisms available. Senile macula degeneration would be an example, though perhaps the rate of degeneration might be slowed.

The more important question is not whether homeopathy has a role, but what role does homeopathy have in different clinical situations.

THE SUPPORTIVE ROLE

The question is often asked, 'Would you treat acute appendicitis with homeopathy?' or 'Would you treat a heart attack?' The answer is 'Yes and no'. We might ask, 'Would you treat a heart attack with Aspirin?' The answer is 'Yes and no', and for the same reason. Aspirin has an important contribution to make. We would now be negligent not to give it. But it is not by itself the proper management. This is the way to regard the role of homeopathy in many acute situations that require emergency care.

The supportive role for homeopathy is extensive. The use of Arnica in pre- and postoperative and antenatal care and childbirth has been mentioned, as has the palliative role of homeopathy in terminal care and in mitigating the adverse effects of radiotherapy and chemotherapy. I have a particular interest in using homeopathy in the physical and behavioural symptoms of all forms of learning disability. In situations such as these we are integrating homeopathy into care in exactly the same way as we integrate a variety of conventional management options. The role of homeopathy is in many cases supportive to other interventions, and in no sense alternative.

COMBINING HOMEOPATHY AND CONVENTIONAL MEDICATION

There is no reason why homeopathic medicines and conventional drugs should not be combined in the one regime. It is inexcusable for conventional clinicians to tell patients that they cannot or will not continue to treat them if they are receiving homeopathy; that it is 'either/or'. The two methods are not mutually exclusive, and ignorance is no excuse because a telephone call would resolve the issue. It is equally inexcusable for homeopaths to tell patients they must stop taking their conventional medication if they want to benefit from homeopathy. When a patient is receiving conventional medication then homeopathy has two aims: to achieve improvement in the condition over and above what has been achieved with conventional medication, and to make the patient less dependent on or independent of conventional drugs. When their progress justifies it these can be carefully withdrawn.

There are situations where homeopathy cannot influence the condition in the presence of the conventional drug. These are where natural physiological function has been taken over by the drug and so cannot be enhanced or modified by any other stimulus. The obvious example is the control of menstrual disorder by hormone preparations that suppress physiological control. This is not the case, however, in the treatment of hypertension where the conventional regime has already produced a normotensive state. Because homeopathy is treating the whole person and the whole clinical picture, and because blood pressure is a multifactorial phenomenon, adjustments other than those produced by the hypotensive drug may occur. In this case the blood pressure will fall further, and reduction in the dose of the hypotensive will be necessary. This requires collaboration between the doctors or practitioners concerned. It also requires the homeopath to be alert to this possibility if the patient presents with some other problem. This is an example of the situation described earlier in which the patient inadvertently withholds essential clinical information because they take it so much for granted. Maintenance treatment is such a routine part of life for patients with long-standing and well-controlled hypertension that they may very well not mention it, and even a referring doctor may omit to do so. Given the right prescription, homeopathy may affect the whole clinical picture even if part of it is not revealed. If that part is a medically suppressed hypertension, a further physiological lowering of the blood pressure might be undesirable.

Such an event could be regarded as an adverse interaction between the conventional and homeopathic medication. In fact it is only adverse if it is unforeseen. If anticipated and allowed for by careful monitoring it is, of course, entirely beneficial. This is a situation where the physiological response to homeopathy and the action of the conventional drug are cumulative. Another example would be the treatment of diabetes, where lowering the blood sugar with homeopathy might destabilize the control if all concerned were not alert to the possibility.

Homeopathic treatment can undoubtedly be more difficult in patients who are on conventional regimes of long duration or multiple conventional drugs. This is not a reason for withdrawing any medication unless it is ill judged and excessive. It does require patience and perseverance, and tailoring the homeopathic regime to the situation. It is often claimed that steroids inhibit the action of homeopathic medicines. I have never found this to be the case and others concur.

FIRST CHOICE HOMEOPATHY

There are many conditions that are not emergencies where homeopathy would be appropriate as a first choice treatment. Most present in general practice, which would be the ideal setting for homeopathy if the time and the expertise were available. Early referral for homeopathy, which can make such a difference to outcome, is usually not an option. Even if an NHS clinic is available and accessible, many waiting lists are too long, and most people cannot afford private treatment even if it is available near at hand. The only people who do have an option are fundholding GPs who have a skilled homeopath working nearby. Patients who have a well-trained homeopathic GP are very lucky.

A limited list of amenable conditions includes:

1. Children – these respond extremely well to homeopathy for

commonplace ailments and the early episodes of conditions that often become recurrent with conventional treatment: catarrhal conditions, otitis, glue ear, tonsillitis, conjunctivitis, respiratory infections.
2. First aid and minor trauma.
3. Self-limiting illnesses, which account for the consumption of so many analgesics and antibiotics.
4. Infections that may not be self-limiting but where the avoidance of antibiotics would be desirable.
5. Allergies and dietary intolerance.
6. Irritable bowel and similar psychosomatic disorders.
7. Migraine and chronic headache.
8. The *onset* of insidiously progressive conditions such as rheumatoid arthritis, eczema and other skin disorders, asthma.

This is not a list of conditions that are always easy to treat, but of conditions where homeopathy can have a major role if introduced early enough. Concurrent conventional treatment may be necessary, for example in asthma. In general practice it is feasible to develop protocols to assist the treatment of many of these conditions within the constraints of time and this possibility is being actively researched (Reilly D 1996 unpublished work, Smulders M 1996 awaiting publication).

BOUNDARIES OF COMPETENCE

Circumstances will often determine whether homeopathic treatment is feasible – time in general practice, cost, access to the patient or the practitioner, the knowledge and good will of other clinicians involved, and so on. Competence and circumstances may interact to affect the decision to treat either way. In private practice, for example, we may decide not to treat patients who live too far away to permit regular follow-up, or conditions that require a level of availability that we cannot provide. If we see a patient with otitis media in general practice the decision whether to use homeopathy might depend on some permutation of the time available to assess the patient, confidence in our ability to choose the right prescription, the opportunity to follow up the patient closely enough, the willingness of the patient for homeopathy and their tolerance of the management plan.

Confidence in our ability to choose the right prescription depends, as with the exercise of any skill, on our level of knowledge and experience. Competence involves awareness of the limits of our expertise. Within these limits, however modest they may be, we can be extremely competent; beyond them we become incompetent. It is a matter of driving within the limit of our lights. It requires the same kind of professional judgement and discipline as in any area of medicine; that is, whether, when and how to intervene with any of our repertoire of skills in particular situations and with particular patients. The exercise of this judgement is no different in homeopathy to the rest of medicine.

The discussion of perspectives and strategic options in other chapters gives an indication of the possible complexity of some cases and the level of knowledge and experience required to use homeopathy effectively in all cases. In fact even the most experienced of us are often stuck; aware that our failure to achieve any benefit for the patient is the result of our own limitations rather than any other obstacle. Paradoxically, however, it is possible for a relative beginner to achieve success in a difficult case because the patient concerned presents an example of some particular insight or piece of knowledge that he or she has already acquired. Beginners are well advised to treat what they already know rather than the patient who arouses their therapeutic enthusiasm. That means applying the knowledge they have acquired when they see a clear example of it in the patient in front of them, rather than deciding to treat a patient and then trying to acquire the knowledge to do so. Of course, as already implied, and as is true for all clinicians whatever their experience, we will always be confronted with patients for whose benefit we will need to acquire more knowledge than we already have. Similarly we all learn by working at the edge of our competence, pushing ourselves to extend the limits of our knowledge and experience to be able to respond to greater challenges. This process of learning by experience makes supervision extremely important, and supervision of the learning experience is probably inadequate in most medical training, including homeopathy.

In general practice, where most doctors in the UK begin to practise homeopathy, the opportunity exists to study as you work, to treat when you see what you know and to use appropriate clinical strategies and protocols. We can fall back on conventional treatments when we do not know enough, or adopt a belt and braces approach. This is a very satisfactory process, whose horizon is limited only by the lack of opportunity to spend an increasing amount of time, both in study and with those patients who require it. This makes it difficult for GPs to acquire the depth of knowledge that will make it possible to treat the whole spectrum of patients and morbidity.

Most doctors in the UK who wish to develop their homeopathic skills for this purpose turn to consultant work, often in private practice because openings for specialist practice within the NHS are so few. Here they have to rise to the occasion. It is difficult to tell a private patient at the end of the first consultation that you are not sure if you can cope! Even experienced practitioners will often put in literally hours of homework to analyse the case and select the prescription. Fortunately the therapeutic virtues of a good homeopathic consultation, which have been discussed earlier, will do a lot to sustain the patient while waiting for the prescription.

The lack of exposure to large numbers of patients before and during their homeopathic training is an obvious problem for NMQP homeopaths, most of whom are highly professional and whose knowledge of homeopathy may be superior to that of many of their medical counterparts. There are a number of issues concerning the boundaries of competence of NMQP homeopaths that are beyond the scope of this book, most obviously questions of diagnostic skill and general clinical management. Suffice it to say that I believe they can be resolved to the satisfaction of all concerned and in particular to the benefit of patient care. It is almost certainly not feasible to provide the best quality homeopathy to all who may require it in years to come without integrating the work of NMQP homeopaths and doctors.

In essence the question of acquiring competence in homeopathy is no different from the same issue in any branch of medical training; consequently the questions of who treats what are very similar. One possible difference, however, is that the complexity of the case cannot be so easily judged from the nature of the morbidity as in conventional medicine. Although GPs become used to uncovering complex dynamics beneath the surface of apparently minor or major problems, by the time they reach secondary care patients can be more readily allocated on a complexity : experience basis. In homeopathy 'trivial' and commonplace morbidity, like chronic catarrh, can have complex dynamics that require appropriate expertise.

One of the dangers of OTC sale of homeopathic medicines is that it gives the impression that treatment of many conditions with homeopathy is a largely DIY affair that can be mugged up by anyone reasonably intelligent from a suitable book. This is no more true than the inference that the OTC availability of hydro-cortisone cream makes dermatologists redundant. (Though the widespread availability of skilled homeopathy might thin their ranks!) First aid homeopathy in the home is very valuable. For serious, established or recurrent illness special skills are required.

DIFFICULT CASES AND DIFFICULT PATIENTS

It is already apparent from what has been said that the ease and difficulty of treatment in homeopathy cannot be categorized easily or consistently. Two patients that powerfully influenced my interest in homeopathy were potentially difficult cases seen in the same week who improved dramatically after one prescription made in the course of routine GP consultations. The prescription was the same in each case, and was possible because I had the book open at the appropriate page on my desk. Beginning at 'A' I had reached the materia medica of the homeopathic preparation of Aluminium. The first patient was an 8-year-old girl with megacolon, radiologically proven and under the care of a paediatrician. Her life was a misery, as much because of the huge quantities of lactulose she was taking to stimulate bowel function as anything else. Her symptoms had all the characteristics of Aluminium that I had just been reading, and the results of the prescription astonished me. She required no more lactulose after a few days, and I think only two more occasional doses of Aluminium. I was able to follow her up for 5 years with no more problems. The other patient had general weakness and malaise and vasodynamic problems in the legs unresolved despite lumbar sympathectomy. These, too, resolved with homeopathic Aluminium, whose clinical picture they matched. It was particularly interesting that on reading the name of the medicine the patient recalled that during the war she had worked in a munitions factory where the atmosphere was constantly polluted with aluminium dust. Whether the anecdotes impress you or not the experience certainly impressed me, but the point is that two challenging cases were successfully and easily treated, largely by serendipity.

Some cases are always difficult or beyond the scope of homeopathy. Severe endocrine and major deficiency disorders have been mentioned already. Major neurological disorders and cancers seldom show more than a palliative response, though it is difficult to know if the rate of progression has been slowed. Some homeopaths claim consistently good results in neurological disorders and many report occasional excellent results, but we should be highly circumspect about the possibilities of improvement. The difficulty of healing long-standing chronic diseases that have received continuing substantial or multiple conventional medication has also been mentioned. Conditions with a deeply entrenched family history can be difficult to treat – a high incidence of early cardiovascular death, for example. Psychotic and other severe mental illness obviously require great care and experience. Their difficulties often arise from problems of general management as much as from their inherent clinical characteristics. There are many well-indicated medicines for their treatment. Homeopathy has a potentially important role in psychiatry.

Quoting disorders like this, however, is misleading because it is often not so much a matter of difficult disorders as difficult patients. The whole thrust of the preceding chapters has been the different dynamics of individual illness. It is not the pathology per se that is necessarily the problem but the number of levels or layers of illness, or the nature of its evolution, the interplay of multiple aetiological factors for example. It is a great mistake to make the nature of the pathology a sole indicator for the expectation of outcome. It is only in the context of the whole picture that these things can be judged, sometimes only in the context of the response to the early stages of treatment, or in the light of the 'obstacles to cure' that may reveal themselves. These factors are discussed in the next two chapters. The title of one of the best-known contemporary books on homeopathy was originally 'The patient not the cure' (Blackie 1976, later called 'The challenge of homeopathy'). It evokes the extraordinary individuality of the patient who is ill and of the illness that patient presents. The difficulty of treatment can in the end be assessed only in this light.

Key points

- Homeopathy is an appropriate treatment in many different clinical contexts, from domestic and first aid use to complex conditions requiring specialist expertise.
- Its potential in different settings requires more extensive investigation and demonstration.
- Collaborative care will greatly assist this process of evaluation.
- Homeopathy and conventional treatment are not mutually exclusive. They can be effectively integrated and truly complementary to one another.
- The integration of homeopathic and conventional regimes requires careful management.
- Competence in the use of homeopathy depends on the interaction of morbidity, circumstance and expertise.
- The scope of homeopathy is determined by the capacity of the organism's self-regulating mechanisms to respond to the disorder.
- The complexity and the possibilities of homeopathic treatment depend upon the dynamics of the illness in the individual patient rather than the pathology alone.

REFERENCES

Blackie M 1976 The patient not the cure. Macdonald and James, London
British Medical Association 1986 Alternative therapy. British Medical Association, London
British Medical Association 1993 Complementary medicine. New approaches to good practice. Oxford University Press, Oxford
Erp V, Brands M 1996 Homeopathic treatment of Malaria in Ghana. Open study and clinical trial. British Homeopathic Journal 85: 66–70
Gaucher C, Jeulin D, Peycru P, Pla A, Amengual C 1993 Cholera and homeopathic medicine. British Homeopathic Journal 82: 155–163
Jacobs J, Jimenez L, Gloyd S 1993 Homeopathic treatment of acute childhood diarrhoea. British Homeopathic Journal 82: 83–86
Jacobs J, Jimenez L, Gloyd S, Gale J, Crothers D 1994 Treatment of acute childhood diarrhoea with homeopathic medicine: a randomized clinical trial in Nicaragua. Paediatrics 93: 719–725
Reilly D, Taylor M 1993 The postgraduate experiment. In: Developing integrated medicine. Complementary Therapies in Medicine 1(Suppl 1): 29–31
Swayne J 1989 Survey of the use of homeopathic medicine in the UK health system. Journal of the Royal College of General Practitioners 39: 503–506
Swayne J 1990 Thinking what we are doing. British Homeopathic Journal 79: 82–99

9

Treatment strategy

Although particular treatments have been mentioned to illustrate certain topics, this is not a book about therapeutic method. It lays a foundation for therapy by discussing the information we need to treat the patient: how to elicit it, the conceptual framework for it, and the rationale for treatment that it provides. This account will be completed by considering these same aspects of the response to treatment in Chapter 10. At this stage, though, we need to draw together the themes of preceding chapters to show how they will contribute to the treatment strategy. The following review recapitulates many points made earlier within a general strategic framework, but provides only an introduction to the subject.

STRATEGIC OPTIONS

The preceding chapters have broadly identified three types of prescription: those based on the presenting problem, those based on a view of the patient as a whole and those based on the wider context of current clinical picture (Fig. 9.1).

Problem-based prescriptions

These represent a circumscribed view of the clinical state. The prescription corresponds to the local and particular characteristics of the presenting problem. It may be a known 'specific' for that problem. Its correspondence may be based on the pathology

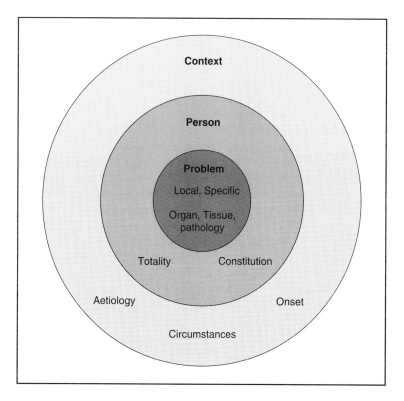

Figure 9.1 Strategic options: problem based, person based and context based.

or an affinity for the tissue or organ involved. It does not take account of coexisting disorders or of the more general characteristics of the individual.

Whole person prescriptions

These are prescriptions based on the totality of the symptoms at the time, or on constitutional characteristics independent of the symptomatology. The totality should subsume the key symptoms of the presenting problem. The constitutional features should be consistent with the clinical picture unless the constitutional prescription is to be given between episodes when there are no active symptoms.

Context-based prescriptions

These are prescriptions that reflect the circumstances out of which the current clinical picture has emerged. They are the predisposing and provoking factors in the patient's medical or social history, lifestyle or relationships. They include exposure to specific toxic or pathogenic agents – poisons, drugs, organisms, allergens, etc. These indications may point to the same medicine as the problem-based or whole person prescription. For example, the patient whose history of psychological trauma suggests a role for Staphysagria in the treatment strategy may also present the clinical picture of Staphysagria in their symptomatology. Alternatively the indicated medicine may be quite different. An example would be the isopathic nosode in a patient never well since a past illness such as brucellosis.

PERMUTATIONS

There are many factors that influence the choice of strategic option, but in some clinical situations any one of these three types of prescription may be appropriate. In a patient with hay fever, for example, the prescription might be based on the local symptoms in the eyes and nose, or the wider totality, or, preseasonally in the asymptomatic patient, on the constitution, or an isopathic preparation of pollens may be used. Similarly, it is entirely appropriate to use a local prescription to treat the circumscribed features of one disorder in a patient with chronic illness and multiple problems. A comprehensive approach to the whole spectrum of disorder might be the ideal, but relief of one symptom may be the pragmatic best that the circumstances permit. In another case the local prescription for the acute episodes may not prevent recurrence but may be invaluable for palliative use while a broader-focused preventive or curative regime is developed.

Different strategic permutations can be applied in many clinical situations (Fig. 9.2), and it cannot be said that any one is necessarily best. There are arguments for and against particular strategies in particular situations. These will be resolved only by research, if and when that becomes feasible.

The following sections discuss some of the strategic considerations that arise in certain clinical situations.

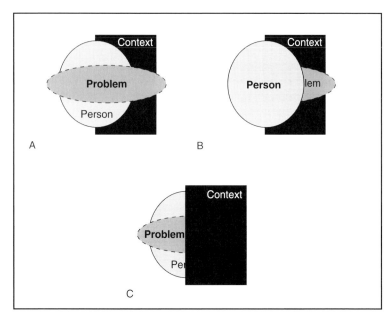

Figure 9.2 Permutations: problem-, person- and context-based views.

PREVENTION AND PROPHYLAXIS
Prophylaxis of predictable stress and damage

These stresses may be physical (including environmental) or psychological. The value of homeopathy to support surgery and childbirth has been mentioned. It can be used similarly to mitigate the effects of sporting activities – muscle, tendon and ligament strains, stiffness and contact injuries. Environmental situations where prophylaxis is effective include exposure to cold, altitude sickness and travel sickness. Prevention of allergic reactions could be included under this heading. Homeopathy is frequently used to mitigate emotional stresses such as driving tests, exams and public speaking. The first homeopathic prescription that I followed was the advice of an experienced GP homeopath to take homeopathic Coffea (coffee) before setting out on a night call and on returning to bed after it. This is an excellent prophylactic for the overactivity of mind that prevents sleep in many situations.

Promoting health

Some stresses are unavoidable consequences of some activities. We can reduce our vulnerability to sporting injury by increasing our fitness, but this will not prevent us from getting hurt. There are situations of challenge of various kinds where it is natural and normal to feel anxiety. Nevertheless, to some extent our need for prophylaxis is a measure of our susceptibility. If we can reduce this susceptibility by remedying the constitutional or familial traits that give rise to it so much the better. The anxiety or the susceptibility to cold, which require prophylaxis in particular circumstances, are likely to be habitual characteristics of the individual – perhaps not of a degree to cause problems at other times, but distinctive none the less. Treating this susceptibility may avoid the acute problem.

Patients who are familiar with homeopathy will sometimes ask for constitutional treatment for health promotion for themselves or their children. This is a legitimate request. In fact, as the consultation proceeds it usually emerges that they are not wholly symptom free, and almost certainly have a past history or family history indicating some vulnerable trait. In addition there will be characteristics of physical constitution or personality that are distinctive. These may be normal in the sense that they are within the normal range of experience, or in the sense that the patient accepts them as part of their nature without complaint, but they may well be distinctive enough to provide a constitutional picture. Where there is a personal or family history that predisposes to future illness, this approach is obviously particularly desirable. Prenatal treatment can be prescribed in the same way. It is beneficial for the mother and, it is believed, the child.

The assumed benefits to the child from prenatal treatment are obviously wholly speculative. It would require the most elaborate study to investigate, and the informed empiricism of the clinician cannot assist in making a reliable judgement in this situation. The same applies to another proposition about the ability of homeopathy to promote future health. This is that its use will, almost by definition, improve the healthfulness of the individual. The response to treatment implies that the body's own ability to cope is enhanced by homeopathy, and its susceptibility to illness reduced. The corollary is that this enhanced resourcefulness or reduced susceptibility confers lasting benefit, some degree at least of increased healthfulness. When medicine as a whole has greater confidence in the general efficacy of homeopathy, this will be a proposition worth investigating. One small step has been taken in this direction by the inclusion of questions about the use of homeopathy in the Avon Longitudinal Study of Pregnancy and Childhood (ALSPAC), 'Children of the nineties' (Golding 1996). It is difficult to predict what data this will yield or how reliable they will be, but it may provide some insight into the health promotion benefit of homeopathy.

ACUTE ILLNESS

This is the most straightforward clinical challenge in homeopathy. The indications are vivid because of the acuteness of the illness. Their individuality is usually distinctive if the totality of the symptoms is considered, but the local symptoms (the detailed characteristics of the sore throat, gastroenteritis, etc.) may be sufficient in themselves. The challenge is straightforward because other dimensions do not enter into it. The focus is on the local symptoms and signs or the totality. The 'shift in the way we view our work' may need to be only very small to accommodate the additional information necessary to the homeopathic prescription.

Because it is straightforward does not mean it is easy, however. One of my first courses as a GP homeopath dealt with upper respiratory tract conditions. It presented a multitude of possible medicines for every permutation of symptoms. On returning to the practice, at the end of February, I was confronted by just such a profusion of symptomatology. The impossibility of achieving the necessary pattern recognition in every case severely dented my enthusiasm. This was bad teaching. A few prevalent symptom patterns should have been identified and taught with a consequently higher expectation of success in a few patients. This is now the trend in GP teaching. The use of protocols has been mentioned. These can be designed to identify the few medicines whose local symptoms or totality may encompass perhaps two-thirds of the clinical pictures of a particular acute syndrome. Specialist homeopaths will expect to do better, but will see fewer acute patients and may lack the clinical experience to reinforce their learning.

There are some acute situations where the clinical indications are much the same from one patient to the next and the choice of prescription is quite restricted or specific. Arnica prescribed for trauma was the most common prescription in general practice in the survey referred to above for that simple reason (Swayne 1989). Acute epidemics may present a small number of dominant clinical pictures. Once these have been identified the choice of prescription for individual patients is simplified.

Recurrent acute illness; episodic illnesses

If acute episodes respond to homeopathy but recur, the acute prescription has obviously not affected the patient deeply enough to remedy the underlying susceptibility. A wider (totality or constitutional) or deeper (historical or aetiological) perspective will be required to develop the treatment strategy.

Acute exacerbation of chronic illness

This may respond to the medicine already prescribed for the underlying complaint if the clinical picture of the exacerbation corresponds. If not, the appropriate similimum for the acute phase will be required. In this situation, however, we may need to distinguish between an exacerbation in the natural course of the disease and a treatment aggravation. This phenomenon has been mentioned already and will be discussed again in the next chapter. If the exacerbation is the result of a first phase therapeutic response it will have a relation in time to the administration of the medicine. It may also be better tolerated by the patient than an exacerbation would normally be. If the conclusion is that this is a therapeutic aggravation, it is as well to allow it to run its course without intervention if it is safe to do so and the patient can tolerate it. If not, conventional treatment sufficient to make the exacerbation tolerable until it passes is usually recommended rather than using another homeopathic prescription while the response to the last is still progressing. A therapeutic aggravation will lead to some improvement in the chronic state.

Intercurrent acute illnesses during chronic illness

Here again the significance of the acute episode needs to be assessed in the context of any homeopathic treatment of the chronic illness. Changes resulting from treatment, such as syndrome shift and the return of old symptoms, must be distinguished from new intercurrent episodes. Changes arising from a previous prescription that indicate a favourable response should not be interfered with if at all possible. If they do require intervention, once again palliative conventional treatment may be preferable to homeopathy. There is debate about whether the use of the homeopathic medicine appropriate to this acute state enhances or inhibits the general progress of the patient if it is a self-limiting phase in the progress of the therapeutic response.

Where the acute illness is not part of the therapeutic evolution of the chronic state it will nevertheless be a related manifestation of the fundamental state of the patient, a related facet of the whole. The sensible and pragmatic course is to treat it with the medicine that corresponds to the clinical picture at the time because that is what the patient evidently needs. But it should also be studied for the insight that it offers into the treatment of the chronic state. The acute illness may illuminate aspects of the case that were previously unclear and change our perception of the pattern as a whole.

CHRONIC AND PERSISTENT ILLNESS

This heading is chosen to include not just patients who have a specific chronic disorder such as multiple sclerosis, rheumatoid arthritis or asthma, but those who are persistently or frequently ill with different complaints that develop in sequence or alternate over a period of time. This development or alternation may itself be characteristic of the pathogenesis and behaviour of conditions in the materia medica of a particular medicine (Box 9.1).

The treatment of chronic and persistent illness may be a matter of one well-chosen prescription, or it may require years of patient and painstaking work that uses all the perspectives and possibilities of treatment described in previous chapters. The question as to what extent we can predict response and progress will be dealt with in a later section (see Expectations, p. 166). The focus of our prescriptions may be influenced by this. In terminal

Box 9.1 Alternating symptom patterns*	
Impaired hearing alternating with eye symptoms	Guarea
Toothache alternating with itching in ear	Agaricus
Abdominal pain alternating with headache	Cina, Plumbum
Rheumatism alternating with diarrhoea	*Kali bichromium*, Dulcamara, Cimicifuga
Vaginal discharge alternating with nasal catarrh	Kali carbonicum
Asthma alternating with eruptions	*Sulphur, Hepar Kalmia* (+ 5)
Bronchitis alternating with diarrhoea	Senega
Pain in the shoulder alternating with pain in the hip	Kalmia

*Type indicates repertory grades.

care, for an obvious example, our palliative intentions are likely to be best served by local prescriptions or the possibly limited totality that best represents the patient's most pressing needs.

Treatment strategy in chronic illness can be based on the following principles:

1. To respond appropriately and faithfully to the need expressed by the patient
2. To work within the scope of the patient's aspirations and insights
3. To recognize the constraints of the circumstances and our own competence and work within these
4. To consider the need for other expertise or for other forms of treatment.

Responding appropriately to the patient's need

In all medicine we should seek to do this by coming to an understanding with the patient about their need, and in helping the patient to come to an understanding with themselves. In a story by Kafka (1949) a country doctor says, 'To write prescriptions is easy, but to come to an understanding with people is hard.' To help people come to an understanding with themselves is harder still. But these hard tasks must accompany the writing of prescriptions or the performance of procedures. If successful they may avoid the necessity for the prescription, as in the case of the patient with guttate psoriasis (p. 136). In every case they will ensure its appropriateness and reinforce its value. In homeopathy the prescription is a reflection of this understanding. The better the understanding we achieve, the more likely we are to make a good prescription, but 'if you understand people you're of use to them whether you can do anything tangible for them or not, for understanding is a creative act in a dimension we do not see' (Gouge 1963).

The specifically appropriate response in homeopathy is the medicine that corresponds best to the need of the patient as expressed in their clinical condition, the presenting clinical picture. This is where we should first focus our attention. The need may be most clearly expressed at a local and pathological level. In that case the prescription will be focused there, as in the patient with lymphoma and a huge spleen (p. 91). Or it may be expressed in the totality of symptoms, possibly encompassing a number of coexisting syndromes.

Other perspectives, recommending other strategic options, will be necessary when clear indications for a prescription are not found in the presenting clinical picture. Then the aetiology or family history may offer another pathway for prescribing. Alternatively, prescriptions soundly based on the clinical picture may fail, or cease to maintain progress. Then again a prescription based on other perspectives of the illness may be needed.

The constitutional picture may help to corroborate the presenting clinical picture. It should not be used to supersede it, but has a supportive role when the clinical picture resolves and a preventive role when used intercurrently in the course of an episodic illness.

In a chronic illness the pattern of indications may change as layers are peeled away. The development of the strategy will be determined by what shows most clearly on the surface at any one time. When we first take the case the different perspectives of the illness may be plainly apparent. A significant family history or aetiology may imply the need for relevant prescriptions at some stage in the treatment. These may prove to be unnecessary in the end because the whole evolution of the illness may be subsumed by the current clinical picture. The medicine indicated by it may pick up all the threads woven into the tapestry of the current illness. When the clinical similimum does not provide the complete answer, the medicines indicated by other perspectives come into play.

There is sometimes a temptation to prescribe first on the basis of a very strong and clear feature of the history that is not encompassed by the clinical picture. Only if it is highly distinctive, and the clinical picture correspondingly vague, should it be given precedence.

The unimportance of symptoms and signs that are common characteristics of the pathology as indications has been emphasized. This should not lead us to disregard the actual pathology itself. As the lymphoma patient exemplified, we must not be distracted by clinical features strongly indicating any medicine whose materia medica does not cover the major pathology. Unfortunately not all reference books are complete and the repertories, which list medicines associated with specific symptoms or pathological states, may not include every relevant medicine, particularly if they are little known. Modern repertories are being continuously updated to remedy these omissions.

Working within the patient's aspirations and insights

When any practitioner sees a patient they may be aware of many dimensions or perspectives of the patient's problem. A GP may be aware of the social, psychological or environmental problems that cause or compound a patient's physical problem. Ideally the doctor may long to promote some change in these that will be conducive to the patient's health. It may be possible to do so, but it may not. Circumstances may prevent it, or lack of resources. But sometimes it is the limitation of the patient's own aspirations or insights that determines the limit of what should be attempted. These cannot be made to coincide with the ideals of the practitioner.

Similarly in homeopathy we may become aware of perspectives of the illness revealed by the history that will require attention if we are to do justice to the problem. We may realize that a local prescription will have only a palliative effect because other dimensions of the patient's health are not encompassed by it. It will not produce the fundamental change that would improve the patient's general well-being. The patient, however, may not wish for a fuller exploration of these other problems. On another occasion the early stages of treatment may relieve the most recent complaint that brought the patient for treatment, leaving more long-standing complaints, possibly well controlled by conventional treatment, unresolved. We may wish to pursue these, but the patient may not.

A variation on this theme arises when the practitioner may have insight into some aspect of the patient's personality or mental or emotional state into which they have none themselves. This insight might recommend a particular homeopathic prescription. To prescribe it when the patient is not ready for it would be wrong and possibly disruptive. It would be similar to imposing an insight in psychotherapy that the patient is not ready to accept. It is possible that the return of the old psychotic symptom in the patient described on page 106 would not have been so acute and distressing if the psychological impact of her adoption had been drawn out more fully and carefully in the consultation before giving the prescription. It may happen that a prescription made on other indications touches upon some psychological aspect of the problem that has not yet been recognized by either patient or practitioner, but we should not deliberately rush in to exploit an insight that has not been properly explored with the patient.

Working within the limits of circumstance and competence

These constraints inevitably affect treatment strategy for any practitioner in any discipline. It is part of our professional responsibility to recognize and adapt to them. The implications are dealt with further in the section on Clinical strategy (p. 163).

Consideration of the need for other expertise or therapy

This, again, is a necessary aspect of professional responsibility. It is also an aspect of clinical strategy. The humility to acknowledge the limitations of our personal skill or our chosen discipline may occasionally fail any of us. This is a particular danger for practitioners of a complementary therapy, who are inclined to be defensive at the best of times. There can be an added reluctance for us to acknowledge difficulty or failure, or the possibility that another therapeutic approach may be better for the patient than ours. But conventional doctors may have the same problem when it comes to yielding their patients to the ministrations of complementary therapists. And professional pride has been known to infect relationships between conventional disciplines.

TREATMENT STRATEGY AND CLINICAL STRATEGY

Treatment strategy is the way we plan a regime for a particular patient. Clinical strategy is the way we decide to deploy our clinical skills and resources for our patients as a whole. A GP homeopath may decide to use homeopathy only within routine surgery consultations, or only in time set aside for longer consultations, or both. The Royal London Hospital provides separate clinics for children, dermatology and rheumatology. Bristol Homeopathic Hospital sees all patients in general clinics. It is arguable that the same skills and knowledge are needed to manage all patients and that segregation is unnecessary; even that it contradicts the whole principle of individualization. On the other hand it is also arguable that particular disease processes do involve particular patterns of therapeutic response and that cumulative experience within specialized clinics will enhance management skills. These choices are a matter of clinical strategy. Their relative merits could be established by careful audit. Many clinical strategies are purely pragmatic.

One of the most important issues of clinical strategy concerns the use of homeopathy in primary care. The elitist attitude regards only those who practise in-depth homeopathy as serious homeopaths. In-depth homeopathy is practised mostly in private practice and in the more leisurely NHS outpatient clinics. Some full-time homeopaths, particularly non-doctors, regard primary care homeopathy of a more superficial kind as meddlesome if not frankly harmful. This is a blinkered point of view. NHS primary care is the setting in which problems most susceptible to homeopathy first present, and in which most chronic disease is managed. It is not and in the foreseeable future cannot be possible to make specialist homeopathic skills available in primary care for all who might benefit from them, even if there were the political will to do so, and even with the involvement of NMPQ homeopaths.

The scope for homeopathy in primary care is enormous, as has previously been shown (Swayne 1989). What is required, and has certainly been lacking in the past, is appropriately tailored training for GP homeopaths focused on an appropriate clinical strategy. This will provide the knowledge and skills to prescribe effectively in most cases of the acute conditions most susceptible to homeopathy. It will provide for the supportive treatment of chronic conditions. And it will also provide for the progressive accumulation of knowledge and skill over time. This will eventually produce a level of expertise that allows GPs to deal with all-comers within their own practice if they have the time and inclination. It will also allow them to work part time in a specialist capacity, as many already do. This programme of training is being pioneered in the academic units of Glasgow Homeopathic Hospital, where already 20% of Scottish GPs have undertaken preliminary training in homeopathy. The ambition is to produce a population of GPs who are experts within the limitations of the clinical strategy for primary care.

The best homeopathic treatment will be the best use of appropriate treatment strategies within the clinical strategies appropriate to the clinical setting. Primary care homeopaths will administer some clinical strategies more effectively than specialists in NHS clinics or private practice because of their opportunities of familiarity, access and availability. They will need the relevant expertise. They will also need the expertise of specialist referral for patients whom their clinical strategies do not accommodate. Specialists will have their own clinical strategies that make best use of their more extensive knowledge of treatment strategies and materia medica, and reflect the constraints of their working life.

SINGLE AND MULTIPLE PRESCRIPTIONS

One of the problems that beset attempts to study homeopathy systematically is the diversity of therapeutic method. One area of diversity is in the use of single or multiple prescriptions in treatment regimes. Brief reference needs to be made to this in the present overview of treatment strategy.

Unicist homeopathy is a treatment method that uses one prescription of a single medicine at a time. No repeat of the medicine, and no new prescription, is given until review of the case specifically indicates it. The single prescription is based on whatever perspective of the case is seen as predominant at the time. If another perspective indicates a different prescription this would never be given in combination with the first prescription, or intercurrently with it. To do so is believed to confuse the issue. It undoubtedly makes it impossible to know which change results from which medicine. This school believes that the progress of the treatment is not best served by such a multiple prescription approach.

Multiple prescriptions take the two forms just mentioned. Combination medicines or complexes include more than one medicine in a single dosage form. This procedure is very similar to the use of combination drugs in conventional therapeutics. A migraine drug may include an ergot alkaloid, an analgesic and an antiemetic. Similarly a complex homeopathic prescription combines medicines with different symptomatic indications relevant to the patient's condition. This method is widely used in France. Such preparations can be bought over the counter in the UK but are seldom prescribed by homeopaths. There are a few exceptions. Some leading doctor homeopaths have had their pet complexes such as Carbo vegetabilis (vegetable carbon) plus Sulphur plus Silica for the treatment of acne. 'ABC', a complex of Aconite, Belladonna and Chamomilla, was once popular for the treatment of fever in children.

The other method of multiple prescribing involves giving separate medicines indicated by different aspects of the symptomatology, or different levels or perspectives of the illness, not in the same dose but intercurrently with one another. For example, a person-based prescription might be given once and followed by regular repetition of the medicine appropriate to particular local symptoms, such as the specific joint symptoms in arthritis. This method intersperses separate and differently indicated medicines in the expectation that they will have a synergistic effect. It is quite widely used in the UK, particularly by doctor homeopaths who have an eclectic and pragmatic approach, adapting their prescribing method to their particular clinical strategy.

There is much debate about the merits and implications of these different methods, but no hard evidence to discriminate between them. That is a necessary task for the future.

EXPECTATIONS

The question of expected outcome is as important in homeopathy as in any other branch of medicine, but in chronic illness is much harder to answer. This is not surprising in view of homeopathy's systems view of illness, its integrative response to the multifactorial nature of illness, and the variety and individuality of the dynamics of illness of which it seeks to take account.

Relevant factors include the sensitivity of the patient. This is not easy to predict but may be revealed by their reaction to other stimuli, including other medicinal stimuli. Another is the vitality of the patient. This is independent of age and type of morbidity. It can be gauged from their spiritual, mental and emotional vigour and the general quality of their body functions. Low sensitivity and low vitality do not indicate an inability to respond to homeopathy, but may require patience, perseverance and/or particular care in prescribing.

The inhibiting effects of long-term use of conventional drugs and conventional polypharmacy on the response to homeopathy have been mentioned. These are not contraindications to homeopathy but may require hard work and patience. A history of medication such as this may be associated with well established and possibly severe organic pathology. Where this is the case the prospect of change is correspondingly limited. The criterion of prognosis is not so much the severity or complexity of the pathology but the resources of the individual to meet the challenge and the dynamics of the disorder. Where the possibility of healing, regulation, compensation or repair exists as part of the organism's natural repertoire of responses to insult or disease we may legitimately hope to stimulate them. Homeopaths can only work this way. If the disease process is not overwhelming, if the vitality is sufficient to respond, we may look to it to do so.

Our expectations will depend upon our assessment of the balance between the apparent resources of the patient to respond on the one hand and the burden of pathology on the other. Our assessment of that burden will be influenced by our knowledge of the dynamic possibilities of the diseased or disordered system, organ or tissue. It will also take account of the effects of conventional medication and the extent to which the patient's circumstances, lifestyle and attitudes are or are not conducive to recovery. This last consideration relates to the need discussed above to work within the aspirations and insights of the patient.

Key points

- Our responsibility as health care professionals is to respond faithfully and appropriately to the needs of the patient. We are guided by the nature of the clinical problem and respect for the patient's integrity and wishes.
- In homeopathy this responsibility must be reflected in the choice of medicines and the strategy with which they are employed. Both must correspond faithfully to the precise evolution and expression of the illness in the individual patient.
- The strategy must be developed in response to the changes observed in the patient after each successive prescription. Although certain elements of the strategy may be foreseen, they cannot be predicted with certainty and must not be assumed.
- In homeopathy, as in other disciplines, treatment strategy will be influenced by clinical strategy. Clinical strategy is influenced by circumstances, the skills of the practitioner and the clinical context within which he or she works.

REFERENCES

Golding J and the ALSPAC study team 1996 Children of the nineties: a resource for assessing the magnitude of long-term effects of prenatal, perinatal and subsequent events. Contemporary Reviews in Obstetrics and Gynaecology 8: 89–92
Gouge E 1963 The scent of water. Hodder and Stoughton, London, p 158
Kafka F 1949 A country doctor. In: In the penal settlement. Secker & Warburg, London
Swayne J 1989 Survey of the use of homeopathic medicine in the UK health system. Journal of the Royal College of General Practitioners 39: 503–506

FURTHER READING

Clarke J 1924, 1925 Case taking, parts 1, 2 and 3. Homeopathic World 59(706): 295–300, 313–318; 60(709): 12–16
Jouanny J 1980 The essential of homeopathic therapeutics. Boiron, Bordeaux
Morrison R 1990, 1991 Methods of case analysis, parts 1, 2 and 3. Journal of the American Institute of Homeopathy 83(3): 63–71; 83(4): 118–125; 84(1): 20–26

The response to the prescription

The changes observed in the patient, and particularly by the patient, in response to the homeopathic prescription are possibly the most intriguing aspect of the whole homeopathic process. Several of these changes have been mentioned already in other contexts, but they will be reviewed systematically in this chapter.

The response to the prescription must not be confused with the outcome of treatment. It is the pattern of change observed in patients in the course of their progress towards whatever outcome is eventually achieved. When it is a well-chosen and effective prescription these changes represent the natural history of the healing process. Because of the absence of any biochemically active component in the medicine we know that the changes we observe are not the product of any direct pharmacological action of a conventional kind. The stimulus is evidently quite different. It is sometimes assumed to be a placebo stimulus. The question whether it is or whether it isn't awaits a conclusive answer, but the balance of evidence is moving against the placebo hypothesis. In either case, however, the changes we observe are valid in themselves. Where they represent a change for the better we are observing the organism's own healing processes at work. As with all medicinal agents, whatever active properties they possess, homeopathic medicines will sometimes act as placebos. As with all good medicine, the whole intervention package – the approach, the consultation, the clinical and therapeutic method – will have a mixture of specific and non-specific effects. When we describe the response to the homeopathic intervention we are describing healing mechanisms at work, whichever aspects of the intervention are responsible. This restatement of the book's recurring theme is the essential perspective within which we must study and criticize the response to the prescription.

In the course of homeopathic treatment the changes that are observed have important implications for the development of the treatment. Their progress over time and their interpretation will determine whether and when the prescription should be repeated or changed, a subject that requires fuller discussion in books dealing specifically with therapeutic method. This account is limited to the present context of case taking, clinical method and natural history. There are two prerequisites. First, the relevant observations will be made only if the information is elicited effectively in the consultation. Secondly, their significance will be fully appreciated only if the record of earlier consultations is sufficiently full and accurate.

PROVING

The experimental pathogenesis of homeopathic medicines, commonly known as proving, investigates the effects of repeated doses of substances in healthy volunteers. These effects are used to identify the pathogenic properties of the substance, and hence its homeopathic therapeutic repertoire: the pattern of disorder that it may be used to treat homeopathically. Together with the study of toxicology and clinical experience, provings provide the materia medica of homeopathic medicines. They can be performed experimentally using natural extracts of the source material, or low or high dilutions of these extracts including dilutions beyond Avogadro's point. Individuals are differently sensitive to the experimental doses, some reacting with markedly greater sensitivity.

In this context we are talking about a similar phenomenon, but produced in patients rather than healthy volunteers, and with regimes that are intended to be therapeutic. Proving symptoms that occur in response to a prescription are distinct from 'aggravations', which will be described next, because they are characteristic of the medicine but not of the patient. They are new symptoms, not part of the clinical picture, provoked by the prescription and characteristic of the drug picture (materia medica) of the medicine prescribed. For example, a patient who medicated herself with Rhus toxicodendron (poison ivy) for rheumatic symptoms in repeated doses over a period of weeks eventually developed the skin eruption characteristic of exposure to poison ivy. The eruption settled when she stopped the medication. The preparation used in this case was a 30C dilution, well beyond Avogadro's point.

This phenomenon is comparable to a conventional drug reaction, except when it occurs in ultramolecular doses. The likelihood of it occurring is related to the sensitivity of the patient but it is not an idiosyncrasy because it is an inherent property of the substance concerned (in fact all substances) to cause such a reaction when administered repetitively in this way.

Proving symptoms can be produced by correct or incorrect prescriptions. They do not often occur, and are almost always the product of excessive or prolonged repetition of the dose. It is possible, however, to obtain a proving reaction from very few doses in an exceptionally sensitive patient. The reaction always subsides when the medication is stopped.

AGGRAVATION

The belief that 'it has to get worse before it gets better' is often associated with homeopathic treatment. This is because of the well-recognized occurrence of an increase in existing symptoms prior to an improvement. It is not, however, inevitable, or at least not to a degree that is recognizable by the patient. The phenomenon is not confined to homeopathy. Some psychological therapies may elicit the same response; so may acupuncture.

The homeopathic principle depends, of course, on the opposing actions of a substance in quantitatively different doses. This is recognized conventionally in the phenomenon of hormesis in which different doses of some substances, within a normally measurable range, exert opposing actions in the organism. In homeopathy the biphasic action results from a single dose. The primary action, as originally described by Hahnemann in paragraph 63 of the Organon, represents the usual pathogenic effect of the substance, exacerbating those features of its drug picture that are present in the patient (Hahnemann & Dudgeon 1982). He postulated that this primary action evokes the secondary or counter-action of the organism's healing processes. The greater the dilution the milder is the primary action. But some degree of primary action, even if subclinical, is believed always to precede the curative counter-action, and in sensitive patients even extremely high dilutions can produce strong primary reactions.

A therapeutic aggravation, consisting of an exacerbation of *existing* symptoms, is the primary phase of the response to the homeopathic prescription. It is not a necessary feature of a good response because as has been said the primary action may be subclinical. When it is observed it is usually a good sign. One possible exception has been mentioned – the reaction to a constitutional prescription that does not match the presenting clinical picture even though it does reflect the patient's underlying constitution.

Another example of such an 'unwanted' aggravation can be provoked by a prescription that is similar, but not closely similar, to the clinical picture; it is similar enough to provoke a primary reaction without stimulating the secondary response. In this case, as with proving symptoms, there are no redeeming features of improvement on any level during or after the event. In fact if there is any dissimilarity between the reaction and the existing clinical picture in the patient it is likely to be a proving rather than an aggravation of any kind, particularly if the dissimilar features are obviously typical of the medicine given.

Definitive criteria of a good therapeutic aggravation are that it involves current symptoms, and that there is some associated improvement in other symptoms or well-being and/or some subsequent improvement in the symptoms concerned themselves.

The time-scale of an aggravation is unpredictable. Its onset can vary from a few minutes to 3 weeks from the prescription. Its duration is from a matter of minutes to, very rarely, a matter of months. An aggravation can be distressing, but once it is identified and explained it is usually tolerated better than the same symptoms would be during an ordinary exacerbation, usually because of some associated improvement in well-being. Where necessary it is better to use the simplest and least possible conventional means to manage the aggravation rather than a new homeopathic prescription.

It cannot be guaranteed that aggravations will be entirely benign, despite their therapeutic potential. If at all severe their management requires appropriate clinical experience and expertise, even if it is in deciding that no action need be taken – particularly, perhaps, when deciding that no action need be taken. Some homeopaths argue that homeopathy is entirely safe. The possible consequences of the provings described above and of some aggravations must, to my mind, be regarded as adverse effects even when the outcome is therapeutic. A sufficiently severe aggravation of bleeding or breathlessness, for example, must be treated as at least potentially threatening until proved otherwise. If there is the least possibility of such a response then appropriate follow-up care must be available. Extensive audit of such events is needed to clarify the situation. Having made this essential proviso, it is nevertheless fair to say that serious aggravations are very rare. Continuing research and development in homeopathic therapeutics are required to eliminate or minimize the possibility of significant aggravation.

In summary then, therapeutic aggravations are the primary phase of a biphasic response to the prescription. They are revealed as such when the secondary phase results in an improvement in the condition of the patient. We know, however, that the placebo response has its counterpart in the 'nocebo' response, when an inert substance provokes a worsening of the condition. In fact research in Glasgow has shown that patients in the same experimental group will show all possible responses to placebo – no change, better, worse (Reilly & Taylor 1993). What is more, they show *different* responses to successive doses (Fig. 10.1).

The research also shows very clearly the influence of expectation on the placebo response, 'no change' being most commonly recorded when administration of the placebo was single blind. In other words the prescriber knew there was no chance of the patient receiving an active preparation. Double-blind placebo doses, where the prescriber knew there was a 50 : 50 chance of the patient receiving the real medicine, most often evoked a distinctive positive or negative response. In other research it has been shown that the effects of drugs in equivalence trials (where all subjects are known to receive an active drug) achieve better results than when tested in placebo-

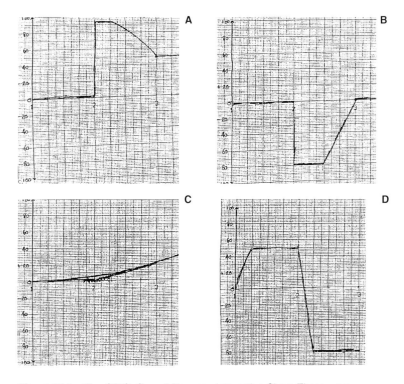

Figure 10.1 The OPIC: Overall Progress Interactive Chart. These were completed interactively by patient and doctor at each monthly visit, so that by the end of the study they had charted the severity of asthma over 12 weeks. On a scale of ± 100% a rise is an improvement, and the line descends where there is a deterioration. Point 1 on the horizontal axis marks the prescription of a single-blind placebo. At point 2, 4 weeks on, the patient has been given, randomized and double blind, either a second placebo or active homeopathy. At point 3 a third prescription is given only if required; of course, those randomized to the placebo group would again receive a placebo treatment. A: No response to the first single-blind placebo. Dramatic improvement within hours to the double-blind randomized prescription – ran a marathon! Waned to 50% within about a month. B: No response to the first single-blind placebo. Dramatic aggravation within hours to the double-blind randomized prescription. 'Worst ever', plus return of old symptoms (rhinitis) and new symptom of midthoracic back pain. C: No response to the first single-blind placebo. A smooth and sustained improvement to the double-blind randomized prescription. D: Marked improvement with the first single-blind placebo. Dramatic aggravation within hours to the double-blind randomized prescription. (From Reilly & Taylor 1993, with permission from Churchill Livingstone)

controlled trials (where one group of subjects receives placebo) (Double 1996). In the first case the level of expectation of a positive outcome is higher than the second where some subjects will not receive an active drug, and the experimenter does not know which.

The Glasgow experiment (see Fig. 10.1) does not, however, show the biphasic response to a *single* dose shown in homeopathy; that is, aggravation and amelioration occur in succession following the one dose. Nevertheless, it may be that placebo can evoke this biphasic response. It will be fascinating to discover to what extent therapeutic aggravation is or is not a feature of both phenomena.

SLEEPINESS

Patients occasionally report extreme sleepiness for a day or two after taking their medicine. This is not the abnormal tiredness or weariness that people may complain of amongst their symptoms. It is a more natural kind of sleepiness such as may follow healthy exertion. It may be disconcerting and inconvenient, but they do not experience it as a malaise. It only occurs in the course of a good response to treatment. There is no certain explanation for this. It is suggested that it is a way of making up for the energy used in responding to the prescription or a necessary part of the healing process.

GETTING BETTER

The fact that people recover from conditions that have hitherto resisted all therapeutic interventions is often remarkable in itself. Practitioners continue to be surprised whatever their theoretical expectations of the potential of homeopathy. Patients use words like dramatic, magic and miracle to describe their experience. Both the degree of improvement and the rate of change can be impressive.

The reason for pointing this out is not enthusiastic hyperbole. It is to emphasize that the quality of response to treatment, whatever the mechanism, so often exceeds our conventional expectations. Or, in other words, the capacity of the mind or body to heal, whatever the stimulus, exceeds our usual expectations. This in turn means that our conventional expectations, and our perception of the mechanisms that underpin them, are clearly deficient. The possibilities are evidently so much greater. Even though we are talking here about response to the prescription rather than eventual outcome, good responses usually do predict good outcome if the case is well managed, and the short-term response certainly suggests the long-term possibilities.

WELL-BEING

This is undoubtedly the most consistently reliable and important indicator of an eventual good outcome, and usually an early response to the correct prescription. It may accompany a therapeutic aggravation, ameliorating any distress or anxiety that may cause. It is a conspicuous variation from patients' experience of the benefit of conventional treatments that may control symptoms but do not necessarily improve well-being. Indeed doctors and patients are only too familiar with treatments that control symptoms but diminish well-being. If that occurs in homeopathy the alleviation of symptoms is no cause for rejoicing. A deterioration of well-being indicates a wrong prescription.

CONSTITUTIONAL CHANGE

Change in characteristics that have previously been considered normal for the individual are another remarkable feature of the response to homeopathy. They often occur early in treatment, may accompany or even precede symptomatic improvement, and usually justify a good prognosis.

In fact the characteristics that change are usually deviations from the norm, which revert towards the norm. They might be regarded as symptoms if they were to arise de novo, but are described as constitutional because they are habitual for that individual. A chilly person may become warmer. A very thirsty person may need to drink less. A craving for salt may diminish. An exceptionally boisterous temperament may become calmer. The mother of an eczematous child of just such a boisterous nature was chiefly delighted at the first follow-up consultation, not because his eczema had improved but because he had become so much easier to live with. There is a type of child whose first act on entering the consulting room is to tip all the toys out on the floor. He (it is most often a boy) then loses interest in them immediately and sets out to wreak havoc elsewhere. Constitutional change can be a blessing for all concerned!

NO CHANGE

No change is of course one possible response to prescription. (This includes continuing deterioration or improvement at the same rate, if that is the current course of the condition.) The first requirement is to ensure that a report of no change really does mean no change. The patient is naturally focused on the presenting complaint and may have overlooked or be unaware of changes in other aspects of their health. Only careful review of the previous notes will reveal this.

If no change is confirmed it means either that the prescription was wrong (and obviously no placebo benefit has occurred either), or that a response to a correct prescription has been blocked by some other factor. This may be an aspect of the evolution of the illness that requires attention before the chosen medicine can elicit a response – perhaps an aetiological factor in the personal or family history, such as in the case of the patient with rosacea quoted earlier (Ch. 7). Or the obstacle may be in the patient's circumstances – medication, lifestyle, relationships, for example. No change does not necessarily imply the failure of homeopathy so much as the need to look further or try harder. Eventually, persistent no change may reveal the failure of homeopathy, or of the homeopath, or for some reason a lack of response to homeopathy in the patient.

INTERCURRENT EVENTS

These will inevitably influence or disguise the response if they have been significantly beneficial or harmful. It is essential to review the possible impact of events when assessing the response, but it may sometimes be impossible to decide the relative effect of the intervention and the intercurrent events. The enjoyment of a holiday, the removal of an anxiety, or improvement in diet or lifestyle, for example, or comparable adverse events, can have an impact that is difficult to distinguish from the effects of treatment or the inherent course of the illness. This is, of course, equally true in any therapeutic setting.

Two other factors are involved in interpreting the presence and absence of change and the influence of intercurrent events. One is the therapeutic vitality of the practitioner, which can be greater or less from time to time. The other is the question of critical timing. Having taken all the various factors that affect a patient's receptiveness and responsiveness to treatment into account, it seems likely that there may be still more subtle factors that determine when an individual will respond best to a particular type of intervention, which it may not be possible to discern.

THE SEQUENCE OF EVENTS AND THE MULTIPLICITY OF CHANGE

It is because of the multifactorial nature of so many changes in health that controlled trials are necessary to test the effect of any single factor. Their limitation and disadvantage are that they are abstractions from reality. By focusing on one mechanism they distract attention from others. This tends to undermine the integrative approach, which is necessary to the proper understanding and management of illness. It is possible that accurate pathography, and closer study of the march of events in the course of illness and healing, might provide us with models of change that discriminate between different processes. Working more assiduously as natural historians might enable us to discern the relative merits of particular components of our interventions. We would not do this by excluding other variables but by observing differences in the pattern of change that result from different sets of variables.

Homeopaths work like this most of the time, using patterns of change to guide them in interpreting the response to prescriptions and in developing the treatment. The sequence of events is an essential part of the pattern. As has been pointed out, this may bear no relationship to the patient's priorities for or expectations of change. Incidental symptoms, well-being or patterns of body function may change before, during or after changes in the presenting complaint. The time-scale of the relationship between these various changes is unpredictable.

As natural historians and scientists as well as clinicians we need to know the significance of this. Conventional drug interventions do not produce these patterns, but how similar or different are placebo responses? As mentioned above, placebo effects are known to be powerfully influenced by expectation. Is the frequent occurrence of *unexpected* change, and change in functions that were not even regarded as disordered, also shown in placebo responses? Or is there a difference between the patterns of response to different subtle stimuli?

This question involves the multiplicity of change as well as the sequence of events – the fact that changes can occur in the symptoms of different syndromes simultaneously. Sequence and concurrence of change are aspects of the same phenomenon. The response to prescription needs to be studied in terms of what changes occur, and in what order these changes take place. The type of change and the sequence of change comprise the overall pattern whose significance we need to understand. It already guides our treatment plan. We need to know what it tells us about the process of healing.

TIME-SCALE

The time-scale of events is unpredictable but it can be plotted. In experiments in my own practice, patients were asked to record the phases of their response to treatment: the period to onset, the period from onset to peak effect, the duration of the peak effect, and the time taken for the response to fade to a plateau. They were surprisingly compliant and surprisingly precise in doing this. They were able to do it for aggravations, for changes in well-being and for improvement in symptoms. The experiment proceeded only far enough to demonstrate its feasibility and did not yield enough data for analysis. It would be possible, however, to accumulate records of the time pattern of change in different clinical contexts (age, morbidity, etc.) and for different interventions. In homeopathy these would include different medicines and different potencies (dilutions). It would, of course, be possible to compare the time patterns of placebo responses with active interventions.

THE 'LAWS OF CURE'; THE DIRECTION OF CURE

A number of observations of the patterns of change that predict a favourable outcome have been formulated as a set of principles known as the 'laws of cure'. They are actually a set of hypotheses derived from empirical observation. Collection of empirical data about these principles is continuing among some groups of homeopaths, but they still need to be rigorously tested. The principles are attributed to Constantin Hering (1800–1880). He was born in Saxony but eventually settled in America where he became inaugural president of the American Institute of Homeopathy. He was interesting for many reasons, including the fact that he took up homeopathy as the result of a commission to write a book discrediting it. In the event his researches led him to the opposite conclusion.

The principles of direction of cure encompass several changes of the kind described in this chapter. They are:

1. Symptoms resolve in the reverse order of their onset, with the more recent first, and the longer established later. The patient described earlier with an aggravation of psoriasis (p. 44) experienced improvement of his more recent arthritis and prostatism first, while his mild long-standing psoriasis got worse.

2. Symptoms recede from above downwards. For example multiple joint pains recede from the upper limbs before the lower limbs. The aggravation of psoriasis just mentioned faded progressively from the scalp to the feet.

3. Symptoms affecting more deep-seated organs or tissues resolve first, and those more superficial later. Asthma must improve before eczema in an atopic patient.

4. The more important organs or systems improve first and the less important later. A heart disorder should improve before a coexisting joint disorder, for example. The relatively greater importance of mental health in this context has been mentioned.

One or more of these changes may be observed in patients who are showing a good response to treatment. But their reliability as prognostic indicators needs to be confirmed. Not all homeopaths are persuaded of their validity. They are a further challenge to our exploration of the dynamics of healing.

RETURN OF OLD SYMPTOMS

Not included in the 'laws of cure' but found to be a similar indicator of improvement in the overall clinical picture is the transient return of old symptoms. The patient whose psychotic symptoms recurred following the treatment of her indigestion was an example given earlier (p. 106). The mechanism and significance of this phenomenon is a matter for speculation, but its occurrence is regularly reported. Sometimes it is apparent that symptoms that recur in this way were originally suppressed by conventional treatment without the underlying cause being identified or resolved. At other times they may be symptoms that seem to have settled spontaneously in the first instance.

It is important to distinguish the reappearance of old symptoms from the appearance of new symptoms. If a prescription provokes new symptoms we conclude that it was wrongly chosen (unless they are quite definitely 'provings' following or accompanying a therapeutic response). Old symptoms whose original occurrence was in the distant past, as may well be the case, and which is not immediately recalled, may be interpreted as new. The possibility must be borne in mind when taking the follow-up history. Similarly the emerging symptoms must be assessed critically so that they are not wrongly identified with old symptoms that were not actually the same.

ELIMINATION

The response to treatment may involve a transient increase in excretory or secretary functions. Sweating, discharges or diarrhoea may increase or arise anew. This is often interpreted by patients as 'getting the poison out of the system'. This may be an approximate explanation but we do not really know what is happening. As with so many of the changes, more systematic observation and data collection are needed as a first step in investigating them further. The transient appearance of a rash is another possibility. It is the transient nature of the symptoms and the context of improvement on other levels that distinguishes them from unwanted new symptoms.

NEW SYMPTOMS

A number of the changes described here may present as new or apparently new symptoms: proving, aggravation of previously trivial symptoms, old symptoms recurring and eliminations. The significance of each is different and important. They must be distinguished from one another, and equally importantly from the results of intercurrent events, and from new manifestations of the progression of the existing disorder that have nothing to do with any event or intervention. This is an important task of differential diagnosis typical of many clinical challenges in applying the homeopathic method, and similar, of course, to diagnostic challenges in conventional medicine.

GETTING WORSE

With the exception of some eliminations, the appearance of truly new symptoms means that the patient is getting worse. This may be because of or in spite of our intervention. The condition may simply be deteriorating, but it will also be apparent that many of the changes described as indicating a favourable response to treatment may proceed in the opposite direction. This negative direction of change may be obvious. On the other hand it may be disguised by other changes that give the appearance of improvement. The parent of a child whose eczema has cleared but who is a little more wheezy may be delighted because the wheeze is easier to manage than the eczema. But this child is getting worse. A patient whose rheumatoid arthritis is better but who has become depressed may be more pleased about the change in the arthritis than concerned about the depression. But that patient is getting worse.

The wrong homeopathic medicine can make a patient worse. It is sometimes stated that homeopathic medicines will have no effect if they are not indicated by the clinical condition of the patient. Earlier in the book the specificity of homeopathic medicines to the needs of the sensitized and receptive patient was discussed (Ch. 1, Homeopathy, natural healing and placebo, p. 2). This exclusivity of the action of particular medicines to particular receptive individuals showing the precise clinical similarity is generally but not absolutely true. It cannot be or we would not see the negative reactions that we do see. These usually resolve spontaneously, but they may take time to do so, and they may be unpleasant enough to require intervention to abort them. Once again it has to be stressed that severe negative reactions are rare, but it is essential to acknowledge the possibility, try to understand it, and seek to avoid it; and to know how to manage it when it happens.

All our clinical knowledge of the possible development of the pathology in the patients we are treating must be applied. This is essential in order to recognize changes that reveal that the pathology is progressing and to permit appropriate changes in management. It is also necessary in order to recognize favourable variations from the predicted course. These may be actual improvements in the condition, or changes that indicate a halt or slowing or mitigation of the progression of the illness even though actual improvement is not possible or has not been achieved.

These possibilities are an important objective of all medical care in terminal or incurable illness. Homeopathy's role in these situations has been mentioned already. It can contribute significantly to the well-being of patients who are getting worse because of the intractable nature of the disease. Clinical observation and judgement are just as important here as in the assessment of potentially curative changes in other cases. The response to each prescription will allow the regime to be tailored to the patient's individual needs, just as the dose of morphine, for example, needs fine tuning to the patient's response to it.

Although discussion of potency regimes has no place here it is appropriate to mention that injudicious use of potencies can worsen the condition of a debilitated patient, in terminal care for example. Increases in the potency (implying power) of a medicine are achieved by serial dilution with succussion (see Glossary). Too high a potency, in other words too powerful a medicine, may seriously weaken the patient. This is assumed to be because the demand it makes on the patient's energies in responding to the prescription is more than they can afford. The patient may in some respects feel better at first if the medicine is correctly chosen, but becomes more debilitated.

DEVELOPING THE REGIME

The response to each prescription – its type, degree, direction and time-scale – will determine how the treatment proceeds. The tactical details of this process belong to a full discussion of therapeutic method, which is beyond the scope of this book. But attentiveness to these changes, and their correct interpretation, is the prerequisite for developing the regime. Good clinical method and good case taking will make good prescribing possible.

CONCLUSION

The processes described in this chapter have been the subject of painstaking observation in millions of patients by homeopaths in many countries for the past 200 years. Nevertheless, collection of data and their analysis have not been systematic enough to define them clearly, to validate them absolutely, nor to tell us all that we need to know about them. We use them to guide our prescribing, but they require far more study if we are to understand the dynamics of the healing process that they seem to demonstrate. The knowledge of them that we do have justifies taking them seriously. Homeopaths need to impress other clinicians and medical scientists with their reality so that the insights into the mechanisms of illness and healing that they offer can be fully exploited.

Response to the prescription: challenges

- The potential of homeopathy to exacerbate disorder, whether in the course of recovery or not, needs to be clearly acknowledged. Its investigation is as important a physiological and clinical challenge as is homeopathy's therapeutic efficacy.
- The incidence and significance of aggravation of symptoms in other therapeutic modalities should be compared with those in homeopathy.
- Detailed study of the sequence and pattern of aggravation and amelioration in response to specific and non-specific therapeutic actions shows every possible permutation. We are far from understanding this phenomenon.
- Throughout medicine we are too cavalier in our attitude to the placebo or non-specific component of all interventions.
- We know that expectation strongly influences the placebo response. Is *unexpected* change a spin-off from this phenomenon, or does it indicate that some other process is at work?
- Accurate pathography may provide us with models of change that discriminate between different responses and different qualities of response.
- Change in habitual, non-symptomatic characteristics of the patient is apparently a commonplace component of the therapeutic process in homeopathy. What are the implications of this in terms of the relationship of the illness or disease process with the whole nature of the patient?
- The detailed sequence and pattern of change in symptomatology is rarely used as a prognostic indicator in conventional therapeutics. What can it tell us about the healing process?
- The time-scale of this sequence and pattern of change can be sensitively and accurately recorded by patients. Its study is therefore feasible and would be fascinating.
- The 'direction of cure', the transient return of old symptoms and the phenomenon of 'elimination' require rigorous documentation and analysis. If they are not a figment of the clinical imagination are they essential features of the natural history of healing?
- The 'differential diagnosis' of change – the discrimination and interpretation of its different patterns – is as important a challenge as is the differential diagnosis of disease.
- The variety and subtlety of responses to the homeopathic prescription, and the questions that they beg, should be more effectively communicated and explored.

REFERENCES

Double D 1996 Placebo controlled trials are needed to provide data on
   effectiveness of active treatment. British Medical Journal 313: 108–109
Hahnemann S, Dudgeon R 1982 Organon of medicine, 5th and 6th edns. Jain,
   New Delhi, pp 73, 79
Reilly D, Taylor M 1993 Developing integrated medicine, part IV. 4. Clinical
   trials: individual patients and their responses. Complementary Therapies in
   Medicine 1(Suppl 1): 26–28

11

Implications

CHALLENGES

Homeopathy challenges us to examine several phenomena that are fundamental to medical practice. These are:

1. Ultramolecular activity. It is currently inconceivable that preparations devoid of any remaining trace of their source material could have any physical or biological activity related to that source material. If homeopathic preparations of this kind are proved conclusively to be active agents, the laws of physics will need to evolve in order to explain the phenomenon.

2. The dose–response phenomenon. The homeopathic *principle* does not depend on the activity of ultramolecular dilutions. At any level of dilution the pathogenic/therapeutic dose–response relationship seems to hold. It is apparently a universal principle that applies to all substances, whether they are naturally pathogenic or not. (Some homeopathic medicines are derived from substances that are inert in their natural state but nevertheless produce an experimental pathogenesis.)

3. Biphasic action. The primary and secondary reactions described in the previous chapter are apparently an essential feature of the response to the homeopathic stimulus. This may or may not be common to other therapeutic modalities.

4. The similimum phenomenon. Unless we are deluded there is a specific and remarkable relationship between the properties of the medicinal substances and the clinical states on which they act. There are now over 3000 homeopathic medicines with specific clinical indications and a repertoire of action in every conceivable permutation of symptomatology.

5. Specific and non-specific effects and placebo. Whether homeopathic medicines are active agents or not the homeopathic approach is a powerful mediator of non-specific therapeutic effects. The process and outcome of homeopathic interventions provide a superb opportunity for the study of the role of specific and non-specific factors in treatment.

6. Disease processes. Homeopathy offers a new perspective of the aetiology and evolution of illness, and the interrelatedness of all its manifestations in one individual over time and at any one time.

7. Natural healing. Since homeopathic medicines, if they are active, can have no conventional pharmacological action, they apparently have their effect by stimulating natural self-regulating and healing mechanisms. The observation of therapeutic change in response to treatment provides us with an unique opportunity to study the natural history of these mechanisms. The same, of course, applies if and when what we are observing are non-specific effects.

All of these deserve the fullest investigation and debate, but it is the last three, with some reference to points 3 and 4, that are the subject of this discussion. The previous chapters have followed two agendas. The first has been to discuss the principles and rationale of the homeopathic approach for students of homeopathy and for others who wish to obtain a broad view of the subject. The second has used this discussion to explore what we may learn about the dynamics of illness and healing from the homeopathic approach. This final chapter draws together the themes of the second agenda and reviews their implications.

OVERVIEW

Broadly speaking all medicine has three roles or functions: as a therapeutic system, as a study of biological processes, and as a social and cultural phenomenon. The focus of these three processes is patient care. Patient care involves the care of communities, of groups such as the family and above all of the individual. Caring about and caring for individuals is the first concern of medical practice. This responsibility to care, which for many is also a vocation, is a personal commitment between the practitioner (including those who provide essential services but may not have direct contact with patients) and the community or individual. It also involves us in activities that as well as having their personal and vocational significance affect our collective work as professions, organizations and members of the medical culture as a whole. These are the science, the philosophy and the politics of medicine. Patient care depends upon them. They sustain it and/or constrain it, according to the culture of the society that provides it. All three of these dimensions of the infrastructure of patient care overlap and interact.

Direct patient care requires a therapeutic relationship, clinical skill, clinical strategy and service provision. By clinical strategy I mean the way we deploy our clinical skills on behalf of individuals or communities. This includes the use of time, the way we decide to direct our skills towards certain people or types of need, the skills we choose to develop, and so on. Service provision involves the way we make ourselves available and accessible to patients.

The science of medicine applies to clinical and diagnostic method, including symptomatology, pathology, epidemiology, molecular biology, genetics – the whole matrix of disciplines concerned to elucidate the nature, aetiology and evolution of illness. It applies to therapeutic method, including prevention, rehabilitation and palliative care. And of course it involves the research method by which we investigate and develop these other activities. All of them involve us in the study of the natural history and complex dynamics of illness and of the healing process. There is an essential trade across their frontiers with the other biological and physical sciences and with sociology and anthropology.

These last two sciences in particular overlap with the philosophical and political dimensions. The philosophy, sociology and anthropology of medicine involve us in the distinction and relationship between sickness, illness and disease. This leads into the question of the relationship between treatment/therapy, healing and holism. And science has its own philosophy concerned with the nature and validity of empiricism, hypothesis, evidence and truth.

The politics of medicine are internal and external. The internal politics determine the role or status of different disciplines and their needs, goals and aspirations. External political forces determine much of what is feasible, often actively directing goals and resources.

The reason for mapping out these various dimensions and elements of medicine is to emphasize that homeopathy is implicated in all of them. Within the scope of its extremely limited resources, it is active in most of them. These limitations involve the small numbers of skilled doctor homeopaths available to meet public demand and to undertake research, lack of clinical provision within the NHS so that even those doctors equipped to provide it are not readily accessible (some health authorities do not purchase homeopathy at all), lack of academic infrastructure, lack of funding for research, and limited representation in the medicopolitical debate. These problems are all interactive, rather like the predicament of the person who cannot get a job because they have no accommodation and cannot get accommodation because they do not have a job.

Homeopathy in the UK is labouring on all these fronts to improve its clinical, academic and service role. Public demand and trial by jury of the population as a whole has ensured that it has become a fact of life in the health care system. Trial by jury of its medical peers still yields an open verdict, although this is an advance on the verdict of 'non-science' that was upheld in years past. Inevitably, and rightly, this verdict will change to 'proven' only when the combination of research and clinical experience achieves sufficient momentum.

PATHOGRAPHY AND HOLOGRAPHY

This book takes for granted that all this work needs to be done, but addresses itself to one particular issue that is generally neglected. This is the importance of homeopathy to the work of pathography and 'holography'. Pathography is drawing or writing the disease process; telling the story of the disease, depicting the disease. Holography is a term we might coin from hologram and holograph for the act of describing the process of making whole or healing.

Pathography and holography, the description and study of the dynamics of illness and healing, are the essential processes of medical practice and medical science. Their virtues were discussed briefly in Chapter 1. In subsequent chapters the observations and perspectives that arise from them have been described, and certain questions and implications highlighted along the way. What are the main themes that emerge?

PLACEBO – WHAT IF IT IS? WHAT IF IT ISN'T?

The wording of this question has been borrowed from David Reilly (1997), whose research has challenged more effectively than any other the proposition that homeopathy is 'merely' placebo (Reilly et al 1994). The balance of formal research evidence is swinging slowly, if not yet conclusively, in favour of homeopathic medicines as active agents. But the point has already been made that proof of the activity of the homeopathic medicines is not essential to the validity of the clinical observations that have been described. Their interpretation and significance do depend in some instances upon what we know about the actual link between the medicine prescribed, its indications and the outcome. In other instances they do not. For example, it is obviously essential to demonstrate conclusively that specific medicines are necessary to stimulate change in specific clinical states (the simillimum principle) if we are to investigate the relationship between the two. If we are to understand *how* the properties of the source material of the medicine relate to the clinical state to which it is homeopathic we need to be sure that the relationship really exists in the first place. On the other hand we do not need to prove the activity of the medicine in order to study the changes alleged to represent the 'laws of cure'. If these changes do accompany and reflect the healing process, their investigation does not depend on the nature of the stimulus that evoked them. If homeopathy is placebo, it presents us with a rich and systematic study of the working of the placebo response, which fully deserves to be taken seriously and investigated. If it is not then the implications are even more startling.

Even if homeopathy is placebo, those of us who use it are still getting results that surpass the ordinary experience of placebo effects in medicine. We have available to us an enhanced placebo of great power and value. The truth of the matter is probably that we are getting the best of both worlds; that homeopathy provides a specific therapeutic tool of remarkable versatility *and* a potent vehicle for the placebo effect. In which case it also provides us with a magnificent opportunity for an investigation of the role of specific and non-specific effects in medicine.

SPECIFIC AND NON-SPECIFIC EFFECTS

The potential of the homeopathic approach to evoke or reinforce a placebo response has been emphasized a number of times already. It is often portrayed as a weakness in homeopathy's argument for therapeutic respectability. It should be regarded as a strength. Whatever our therapeutic method we should seek to maximize the benefit of every aspect of the intervention, specific or non-specific. The non-specific effects of any therapeutic approach are essential to the outcome. They should be enhanced as far as possible. Any approach that uses them to particularly good effect should be particularly valued for what it has to offer and what it has to teach.

Specific effects are usually regarded as those that result from the use of specific therapeutic techniques or agents; these include drugs or procedures we employ. Non-specific effects are produced by aspects of the intervention as a whole that are incidental to these. They include the use of actual placebos, and the 'add on' placebo effect associated with the use of specific techniques and agents. The value of an active drug will include some greater or lesser degree of placebo overlay.

The consultation process mediates most of the non-specific effects that are not placebo components of the active drug or procedure. A GP colleague has identified 35 elements in the consultation that are of potential therapeutic benefit (Hughes-Games J, personal communication). He happens also to be a homeopath, but these therapeutic ingredients are common to all consultations.

We should take it for granted that the outcome of our interventions is always a combination of specific and non-specific effects. In day to day practice it can be difficult or impossible to attribute change to separate aspects of the intervention. It may seem an unnecessary academic question anyway if the patient is getting better. But of course it is necessary if we are to review the justification for and performance of the specific prescription or procedure and develop the treatment accordingly. It is also essential if we are to refine and extend our understanding and use of particular specific and non-specific effects so as to achieve the most effective therapeutic package.

WHEN IS SPECIFIC NON-SPECIFIC?

But here we meet a paradox, or at least a conceptual difficulty. When we deliberately use a non-specific factor of the therapeutic encounter, does it not become specific? The process of paraphrase, which was described in the section Language and meaning (Ch. 4, p. 59), may not only help to clarify the symptomatology. It may also promote new and helpful insights. Paraphrase is a commonly used technique for both these purposes. For some practitioners it will not be a 'technique' but an instinctive and unconscious response to the patient's narrative; it will be part of their non-specific repertoire. For a psychotherapist it will be a specific technique. Thus the distinction between the specific and non-specific elements of a therapeutic encounter will often be a matter of context and usage. The process of case taking in homeopathy, with its necessary detail of enquiry and attentiveness to the patient, is a specific technique whose purpose is an intellectual analysis of the case history in order to identify the indications on which to base a prescribing strategy. It is also therapeutic in its own right. We might say always therapeutic, even in the case of a third party account of the illness in a baby, unconscious person or animal because of the possible indirect effects upon the patient.

An active drug (specific agent) can have an added placebo component (non-specific effect). One clinician's non-specific approach is another's specific technique. This dual effect of various aspects of the interaction between practitioner and patient is common to all medical disciplines. The specific–non-specific dualism is in many instances as artificial and unhelpful as the mind–body dualism that permeates much of medicine. This fact of life does not excuse us from studying and seeking to define and manage the different elements of the specific–non-specific or mind–body continuum appropriately. But we must keep it in mind to prevent us getting the analysis of those different elements out of perspective.

DIFFERENT STIMULUS, SAME EFFECT?

Homeopaths believe that all the changes resulting from the homeopathic intervention can be stimulated by the homeopathic prescription. Even though other factors contribute to a greater or lesser degree to the response in a particular patient, the specific action of the medicine itself is capable of producing the whole gamut of change that is described in numbers of patients collectively. All changes are potentially specific effects. Homeopaths also believe that these effects are achieved by stimulating the organism's own self-regulating and self-healing mechanisms. These are the same mechanisms that are active when the organism responds spontaneously to insult and disorder. They are the same mechanisms that operate whenever that response is stimulated by any external stimulus.

The corollary of this is twofold. First, if they are the same we could not distinguish by observation alone those changes resulting from the specific action of the medicine from those arising from other non-specific elements of the intervention. In fact, if and when the biological activity of homeopathic medicines is proved beyond dispute, comparative studies of homeopathic and placebo/non-specific responses will be necessary to determine whether the two really are the same. We might find homeopathic healing follows a different pathway to other subtle healing stimuli. Secondly, but subject to the same proviso, whatever stimulus is responsible, the changes that ensue are in any case manifestations of the natural healing process.

Whatever the true story of this stimulus–effect relationship waiting to be deciphered, homeopathy presents a close-up examination of the process. Just as a mechanical microscope reveals the healing processes involved in the inflammatory reaction, the homeopathic method provides a clinical microscope with which to examine healing processes in precise detail at a higher level of integration. This is the same microscope as clinicians have used for millennia. In homeopathy it is just employed more assiduously than elsewhere at present.

Until the question of specific and non-specific effects is clarified we cannot interpret with confidence the full significance of all that we observe. Meanwhile we can begin to define the issues.

DISEASE PROCESSES

The following propositions can be derived from the observations described in previous chapters:

Epidemiology

1. *Patterns of disorder in the family history* of an individual predispose to and may predict the pattern of illness they will themselves experience. The familial influence may be multifactorial, and will differ from the inherited traits for single specific disorders whose genetic mechanism is recognized.

If these patterns are a reality this would be confirmed by epidemiological investigation of the association between family history and personal history.

These patterns are identified with certain homeopathic medicines. If the specific action of the medicines associated with them is demonstrated, the recovery of patients from disorders whose history is consistent with the particular familial pattern would corroborate the epidemiological data.

2. *The history of illness during the life of an individual* is the manifestation of a continuous process. All episodes are related to this process over time. At any one time the clinical picture forms a coherent whole. Different syndromes that coexist in the one individual are related parts of this whole.

These clinical pictures, which are effectively discrete epidemiological entities, are identified with specific homeopathic medicines. The identity of these clinical patterns and their consistent occurrence should be susceptible to epidemiological investigation.

The medicines are seen to effect change in any or all of the coexisting syndromes that comprise the pattern.

If their specific effect is confirmed, the response of the patient to their action confirms the reality of the clinical/epidemiological entity so described. If it is not, the fact that separate syndromes change concurrently or sequentially in response to the one stimulus still implies a relationship between them.

3. *Constitutional characteristics* of healthy individuals or of patients in between episodes of illness are associated with a predisposition to certain symptoms and disorders.

The existence of these constitutional types can be investigated epidemiologically (Ives 1981, 1985). The clinical states associated with them could be similarly investigated.

If the specific action of constitutional medicines is demonstrated, the clinical outcome could be used to corroborate the epidemiological data.

4. All these propositions have implications for preventive medicine.

Pathogenesis

1. Toxicology and experimental pathogenesis (provings), as well as study of the natural history of diseases, show the wide variety of systemic disorder that can result from a single pathological cause. This variety is reflected in the observed clinical versatility of the homeopathic medicines derived from the pathogenic agents. These patterns of symptomatology, of coexisting or sequential disorder, are found in patients who have not been exposed to the pathogenic agent concerned. The patterns of coexistence or evolution imply relationships between pathological processes that we often do not understand at present, and may not even recognize.

2. The existence of these patterns is a matter for epidemiological study, as discussed above. Their significance in terms of our understanding of disease processes is an even greater challenge. The descriptive task, the natural history, is the first step.

3. Once proven, the response of these patterns of disorder to specific medicines will help to confirm their coinherence. The experimental pathogenesis of the medicines may then help us to understand the disease processes themselves better.

Aetiology

The relevance of a wide variety of aetiological factors in construing and treating an illness homeopathically has been described (Ch. 7). No systematic study has been made of the association between specific aetiological factors and the types of morbidity attributed to them in homeopathy, as far as I know. This would be interesting. Once again the proven effect of specific medicines associated with specific aetiologies would reinforce the value of the study.

TOTAL PATHOGRAPHY

In many of its treatment strategies, homeopathy seeks a total pathography. It construes the problem comprehensively in terms of family history, personal history, constitution, pathogenesis and aetiology, as a whole. It does this to provide the grounds on which to base prescriptions. In the process it develops a view of the dynamics of illness. This in turn informs the process of case taking and analysis.

This broad schema of pathography is far from being satisfactorily worked out and defined. It contains too much diversity of interpretation, too much unsubstantiated 'doctrine', too much speculation. These are the manifest weaknesses of homeopathy, and they undermine its strengths. Nevertheless this integrative view of illness has its underlying consistency. Better intellectual discipline, better analysis will make it truly useful in informing contemporary perceptions of disease processes. As with many aspects of homeopathy it is a stimulus medicine needs.

HEALING PROCESSES

The inflammatory reaction is one of the fundamental processes of physiological healing. Its components and phases have been painstakingly described, from cellular level to symptomatology. We know that changes in blood supply and white cell activity on one level, and redness, swelling, warmth and pain on another, are all part of it. These are the local tissue changes of the healing reaction.

In its observation of the response to treatment, homeopathy has mapped out a process as intricately orchestrated but on the level of the organism as a whole. The question of whether this process or aspects of it are common to all pathways of self-healing has already been raised. But in any case its manifestations have no counterpart in any conventional account of mechanisms of healing. (They may be reflected in the literature of other complementary therapies that I am not acquainted with.) They are highly distinctive and deserve to be known and investigated by others outside homeopathy. In summary they are:

1. Aggravation: the primary phase of the biphasic response. A therapeutic aggravation of existing symptoms should lead to an improvement.

2. Well-being: this often improves in the early stages of the response. Sometimes it precedes specific symptomatic change. It may improve during aggravation of other specific symptoms.
3. Elimination: this includes discharges, sweating, diarrhoea or rash occurring in the early stages of a positive response.
4. Improvement in multiple symptomatology from one medicine.
5. Improvement in incidental or unconsidered symptoms.
6. Improvement in constitutional traits.
7. Return of old symptoms: transient return of symptoms that had resolved or become dormant at some time in the past.
8. Resolution of symptoms in the reverse order to that of their appearance.
9. Improvement in more important systems before less important (e.g. mind before joints).
10. Improvement in more deep-seated organs before more superficial (e.g. lungs before skin).

These are all well documented in clinical records, but far more systematic recording and analysis are required to provide the basis for further investigation. We need to confirm, clarify and define the changes we observe. We need to examine the relationship of the patterns of healing changes to the disease processes from which they arise. Are particular patterns of family history or pathography associated with particular patterns of healing change? Are particular clinical states more likely than others to show strong primary reactions during treatment? Are particular histories more likely to lead to the return of old symptoms than others? Once proven, the specific efficacy of particular medicines producing particular changes in particular clinical circumstances will provide a tool for investigating these processes in addition to their therapeutic value.

We need also to examine the influence of previous conventional treatment upon the pattern of healing change. Are certain changes more common after long duration of conventional treatment? For example, are skin eruptions more likely to show aggravation after long suppression with steroid preparations? Do allergies respond poorly to homeopathy after previous conventional desensitization?

ONCE PROVEN . . .

This phase has occurred a number of times in this chapter. But the point to which we return time after time is that this proof – the specific efficacy of the homeopathic medicine – is incidental to most of the phenomena described. They are all a matter of empirical observation. Certainly they need to be confirmed and defined by more rigorous collection of data. Either they are valid or they are not. The patterns can be confirmed or contradicted by systematic study. Their validity does not depend on the nature of the intervention. This is obviously true of the disease processes that precede it, but it is also true of the healing processes that follow from it.

The role of the homeopathic medicine is not in any way essential to the reality of these observations, but it does add another dimension to their corroboration and their interpretation. If we consistently reproduce certain patterns of change in certain patterns of illness by use of a specific intervention we have not only a useful therapy but an experimental method. As Professor Harris (mentioned in Ch. 1) said, 'every time we intervene in people's lives we are conducting experiments' (Harris 1989). Every homeopathic case that we take is 'a research project in which we must gather data and reach conclusions' about the dynamics and evolution of the illness. Every time we make a homeopathic prescription we are conducting an experiment in natural healing. Whatever the nature of the intervention, however non-specific the therapeutic effect, we are making this experiment. But if we know for sure that the homeopathic medicine is an active agent in the process, then the nature of the experiment is changed and the conclusions we draw will be different.

Consider the examples of aetiological prescriptions whose results could be explained by psychological or placebo mechanisms (pp. 125–126, 135–136). The aetiological process that such cases exemplify can be studied in their own right. We can investigate whether such and such a family history consistently predisposes to a particular pattern of morbidity; or we might ask whether a certain type of psychological trauma predisposes to a particular illness. The nature of the intervention has nothing to do with it. Similarly we can look for consistent patterns of therapeutic change and study these and their relationship to the particular aetiology, whatever caused the change. If, however, we know that response A is definitely produced by medicine B based on aetiological indication C, we can be that much more systematic in our studies. The phenomenon we are demonstrating has even more far-reaching implications. And, of course, we can apply that rationale of treatment with greater confidence.

Proof of efficacy is not essential to the effectiveness of homeopathy. It will not actually work any better or any worse for it, except in as much as increased expectation will further enhance the placebo component of treatment, as with any medicine. Patients and practitioners will continue to get the same results if it is proven as they did when it was not. More patients will, of course, enjoy the benefits of these results because more doctors will accept homeopathy once its efficacy is proven and more facilities will be provided. Proof of efficacy is not necessary for the study of the phenomena of illness and healing that are identified by the homeopathic method. But proof of efficacy is necessary if we are to achieve the fullest possible understanding of these phenomena, and the fullest development of the therapeutic process.

CONCLUSION

In the famous story, Nelson held his telescope to his blind eye in order to avoid reading the signal he did not wish to obey. Selective deafness or blindness is a convenient ploy in many situations. It is not always so deliberate, of course. As the quotation from Professor Harris in Chapter 1 reminds us, 'What we expect to find is powerfully conditioned by what we have learned. . . . This sets the limits of what we ask our patients about and the extent to which we are prepared to ignore anything they do tell us that is not required by, or does not fit, a pattern with which we are familiar.' (Harris 1989). Propositions become irrelevant or nonsensical, and even tangible objects can become invisible if they have no place within the conceptual framework of our lives or of the task in hand. This is the problem with attitudes to homeopathy.

The first test of a new hypothesis is the extent to which it conforms to, or is a logical development of or a logical departure from, what we already know. Because homeopathy is so far from fulfilling these criteria, contemporary science reasonably demands exceptionally rigorous proof of its propositions. Attention is chiefly focused on the one theme – the dilution of the medicines. In his essay 'Demarcation of the absurd', Peter Skrabenek (1986) wrote 'The absurdity of homeopathy becomes obvious when it is realised that the infinitesimal doses commonly used . . . exceed in dilution the Avogadro number. This means that the homeopathic medicine does not contain even a single molecule of the substance of which it pretends to be a dilution. Truly, "dilutions of grandeur" '. The last phrase is a quotation from another author. He also quotes from 'The comforts of unreason. A study of the motives behind irrational thought' (Crawshay-Williams 1947): 'We must search our mind beforehand to find out what we would like to be true, and having got that clear, constantly discount our natural tendency in that direction.'

So we have to steer a course between the blindness conditioned by what we have learned to expect and the gullibility conditioned by what we would like to find. The latter tendency is why we have to have rigorous methods for testing hypotheses. The former is the reason we need pathographers to provide 'The observation and description of what is before one's eyes, unconditional by preconceived ideas', which 'are the starting point of all scientific research'(Harris 1989).

Proof and pathography

The homeopathic approach is an exercise in pathography. Homeopaths themselves are often unaware of the importance of this role. It is not surprising, therefore, that this function of homeopathy has not been better disciplined, and has not been properly exploited for the insights and research challenges it offers medicine as a whole. This book seeks to remedy the omission by using a study of the homeopathic approach as a vehicle for demonstrating its potential for pathography.

The research potential of pathography is immense. Homeopathy has no prerogative of this, but it exemplifies it. Its clinical method requires it. Pathography is second nature to homeopaths. They have the raw material of research before their eyes and in their case notes. Inevitably its use as the basis of their therapeutic method takes priority and little is done to collate, verify and analyse the material systematically for any research purpose. This must be done, however, if the habitual task of pathography is to yield its full fruits. It must also be done to guard against the distortion of empirical data by preconceived ideas. The tendency to find what we have learned to expect and to look for what we would like to be true is a constant threat.

The inherent validity of the observations we make of illness and healing irrespective of the nature of the therapeutic intervention (subject to the above provisos) has been stressed repeatedly. But so has the absolute importance of the question of the efficacy of the medicines to our full understanding of what we observe.

Significant differences

Consider one last example of this: When different patients suffering the same pathology describe their experience we obtain a number of different clinical pictures. Ten patients with the same disorder may experience 10 different symptom patterns (see Ch. 5, p. 85, Modalities). Why is this, and what does this difference, this individuality mean? Is it just a meaningless accident? Does it have any significance for our understanding of their susceptibility to illness, or their capacity to respond to it effectively? Can we use this information to understand the disease process any better? Does it show any consistent relationship with past history or family history? Does it have any predictive value for the future health of the individual? These are all questions that can be investigated by clinical observation and epidemiological study in any clinical context. They are questions that very few people in medicine are interested in, but they are actually fascinating. The answers to them require systematic pathography.

Homeopathy maintains that these differences are significant – that they are associated with other traits in the individual, other patterns of disorder or susceptibility. It also maintains that these differences reflect particular dynamics in the illness of the individual patient – that it is possible to stimulate or reinforce a favourable resolution of these dynamics with a specific medicine precisely matched to the clinical state of that individual, a medicine that reflects the individual differences. In other words, we can selectively trigger or amplify the healing process with a specific stimulus (the medicine) precisely matched to those individual dynamics.

If this is true it opens the door to a world of new insights into the nature of illness and the healing process. We cannot know for sure that it is true until we have proved conclusively that prescriptions based on the similimum principle have a specific stimulant effect that is *exclusive* to the clinical picture in the individual patient. This proof is not really essential to the therapeutic achievements of homeopathy. Patients will continue to benefit whatever the role of the homeopathic medicine in their recovery. But it is an essential step in the full investigation of the phenomenon that the homeopathic approach describes. It is the essential link between the natural history of the illness and the natural history of the healing process. The description of both of these can be completely valid in itself, because it is based on clinical method independent of any explanatory hypothesis. But our full understanding of the link between them is absolutely dependent on our knowledge of the mechanism that effects the transition. It is essential that we know whether this is the specific effect of the medicine as well as the inevitable non-specific concomitant effects, or whether it is the non-specific effects alone. In either case the pathography is valid and important, but the implications of each alternative are different.

The whole story?

Clinical method in homeopathy, the homeopathic approach, is a richly rewarding and intellectually demanding subject for study. It uses a conceptual framework for observing and interpreting illness and the healing process that differs significantly but not absolutely from the conventional modes. This conceptual framework is based upon pathography, and in its turn provides a structure for the continued practice of pathography. Pathography is the essence of the clinical method in homeopathy. It generates the clinical data on which accurate prescriptions must be based. In the process it continuously generates a wealth of data about the evolution, presentation and natural resolution of illness. If systematically researched these data offer the possibility of new insights into the dynamics of illness and healing.

These possibilities do not depend upon proof of the nature and efficacy of the specific stimulus provided by the homeopathic medicine. They would, however, be greatly enhanced by that proof because it will provide a direct link between the dynamics of the illness, which the medicine represents, and the dynamics of the healing process, which it promotes. This is a challenge whose implications are fully equal to those of the ultimate absurdity of ultramolecular dilution and the fundamental pathogenic–therapeutic paradox of homeopathy.

Finally, and in a sense transcending all these issues, the homeopathic approach acknowledges and affirms the significance and validity of the individual experience of illness and its place in the whole context of the patient's life. In doing this, and if used well, it has its own healing potential – a powerful repertoire of non-specific therapeutic effects. These do not, as is so often implied, undermine the validity of the homeopathic method. On the contrary, they enrich it.

REFERENCES

Crawshay-Williams R 1947 The comforts of unreason. A study of the motives behind irrational thought. Kegan Paul, London
Harris C M 1989 Seeing sunflowers. Journal of the Royal College of General Practitioners 39: 313–319
Ives G 1981 Validation of the homeopathic theory of type. Midlands Homeopathy Research Group Research Newsletter 5: 23–26
Ives G 1985 Constitutional types and homeopathy. Communications British Homeopathy Research Group 13: 11–17
Reilly D, Taylor M, Beattie N et al 1994 Is evidence for homeopathy reproducible? Lancet 334: 1600–1606
Reilly 1997 In: Ernst E, Hahn E (eds) Homeopathy—a critical appraisal. Butterworth Heinemann, Oxford
Skrabenek P 1986 Demarcation of the absurd. Lancet i: 960–961

FURTHER READING

Bellavite P, Signorini A 1995 Homeopathy: a frontier in medical science. North Atlantic Books, Berkely, California
Clover A 1989 Homeopathy reconsidered: a new look at Hahnemann's Organon. Victor Gollancz, London
Doutremepuich C (ed) 1991 Ultra low doses. Taylor & Francis, London
Endler P, Schulte J (eds) 1994 Ultra high dilution: physiology and physics. Kluwer, Dordrecht
Schiff M 1995 The memory of water: homeopathy and the battle of ideas in the new science. Thorsons, London
Vithoulkas G 1979 Homeopathy—medicine of the new man. Thorsons, London

Glossary

Explanations and comments included here are taken from the Dictionary of homoeopathy commissioned by the Homoeopathic Medicine Research Group, supported by Directorate-General XII (Science, Research and Development) of the European Commission. The project was undertaken by the author under the supervision of a steering committee appointed by the Research Group, and in collaboration with leading homeopathic doctors in other member states.

A new and more authoritative dictionary based upon this preliminary work is being developed by the Faculty of Homoeopathy in collaboration with Churchill Livingstone and in consultation with homeopaths around the world, and will be published in 1998. The explanations of concepts given in this version may be subject to revision.

All but one of the definitions given here are original or composed from several sources. The one exception is explicitly acknowledged.

ALLOPATHIC MEDICINE
Treatment that opposes effects of disease

Treatment whose action is directly opposed to or incompatible with the effects of the disease.

Origin. Greek *allos* = other, *patheia* = suffering.

ARNDT–SCHULZ LAW
Dose-related effects

States the relationship between the strength of a stimulus and its effect upon physiological activity; namely that weak stimuli stimulate, moderate stimuli inhibit, and strong stimuli destroy.

AVOGADRO'S NUMBER
Molecular limit of dilution

The Italian professor of mathematical physics Conte di Quaregna e Ceretto Amedeo Avogadro (1776–1856) recognized the connection between the density of gases and their molecular weight in 1811 (Avogadro's theorem). Later on the name of Avogadro became used to state the number of elementary particles in one mole of substance.

1. The number of elementary particles (atoms in elements/molecules in compounds) in one mole of substance. Approx. 6.0023×10^{23} particles per mole.
2. The degree of dilution beyond which no particle of the source material would theoretically exist in the solution – that is, the dilutions C12, or D23.
3. The critical level of dilution depends on various factors, including molecular weight and initial concentration.

BIPHASIC ACTIVITY
Two-phase response

The principle that differences in magnitude of a stimulus on either side of a critical threshold may produce opposite effects (stimulation and inhibition) in a biological system. This phenomenon is exemplified in the Arndt–Schulz Law and in the concept of hormesis.

Compare. Arndt–Schulz law, Dose-dependent reverse effect.

CHRONIC DISEASE
Long-term, deep-seated illness

1. An illness whose onset is usually gradual and whose course is of long duration with no certain prospect of recovery, may consist of recurrent acute episodes, and often involves more than one organ system.
2. In homeopathy, particularly refers to Hahnemann's theory of miasms – Psora, Sycosis and 'Syphilis'.

Comment. The concept of chronic disease has particular significance in homeopathy. Hahnemann attributed the phenomenon to a deep-seated trait in the patient, which he termed 'miasm' and which requires a particular therapeutic approach.

DILUTION
Reduction in concentration

1. Reduction in concentration of a fluid by adding water or other solvent.
2. A stage in the preparation of a homeopathic medicine from its stock or previous dilution (potency) by adding one part to a prescribed number of parts of diluent.

DISEASE AFFINITY
Relationship of drug to disease process

Some homeopathic medicines are particularly associated with specific pathological processes or diseases that occur prominently in their materia medica. For example, bruising and damage to small blood vessels are famously associated with Arnica. This is Arnica's disease affinity.

DOSE-DEPENDENT REVERSE EFFECT
Variant of biphasic activity

The phenomenon in which different dosage levels may produce opposite effects in a biological system.

DYNAMIZATION
Process of imparting therapeutic power

The process through which the biological activity of a homeopathic medicine is enhanced by succussion or trituration.

Comment. See Potentization for discussion of ambiguity in the use of the two terms.

ENTELECHY
Realizing potential

Complete realization and full expression of properties or qualities inherent in a system.

Origin. Greek *en telei ekho* = to be in perfection. Principle expounded by Aristotle.

Comment. Fundamental principle of holism. The action of homeopathic medicines appears to promote entelechy.

ESSENCE
Intrinsic nature

1. All that makes a thing what it is; intrinsic nature.
2. In homeopathy the unique character of a medicine's materia medica; its individuality. Usually expressed in psychological or abstract terms that often reflect metaphorically the physical characteristics.
3. Essential (nuclear) feature that expresses the totality of the patient.

HAHNEMANNIAN DILUTION
Hahnemannian potency

Method originated by Samuel Hahnemann of performing the process of serial dilution in which one part taken from the preparation at the previous stage in the process is added to the requisite number of parts of diluent in a new container at each stage and submitted to succussion (multiglass method). The number of serial dilutions performed in this manner defines the potency according to the proportions (decimal, centesimal, etc.) used in the series.

HEALING
Restoration of health or wholeness

Healing is distinct from cure and treatment because it involves a creative change in the organism towards a state of greater wholeness. Even the healing of a simple laceration demonstrates this, mobilizing latent resources and producing new tissue growth in a way that enhances the competence and strength of the organism. Healing involves Entelechy (q.v.).

Comment. The concept of cure in homeopathy sometimes carries the same meaning given here for healing, but this is not always the case, as when speaking of 'cured symptoms' in a more circumscribed sense.

HERBAL MEDICINE
The medicinal use of plants

1. In its purest form herbal medicine uses extracts of plant material in an unadulterated state – that is, with all the component elements preserved and in their natural combinations and proportions. Cardiac glycosides derived from *Digitalis* are not herbal medicines because they are refined products of the plant. Similarly potencies of Digitalis used in homeopathy are not herbal medicines, although properly prepared the tincture of Digitalis may have both herbal and homeopathic actions.

The emphasis on isolating the active ingredient of drugs of plant origin is a distortion of herbal medicine.

2. Herbal medicines are often considered to act in a more conventionally pharmacological manner than homeopathic medicines, but because of the dependence for the efficacy of

herbal medicines on preserving their complete and unique composition, referred to above, this may not be so.

3. Homeopathy is often confused with herbal medicine because of the plant origin of many of its medicines.

INFINITESIMAL DOSE
Ultrahigh and ultramolecular doses

A generic concept that embraces both ultrahigh and ultramolecular doses; it was used to describe the extreme dilutions introduced by Hahnemann in order to avoid the unwanted effects of primary drug action.

INFORMATION

The properties imparted to the homeopathic medicine by the process of potentization may be described hypothetically as a type of 'information', the 'drug information'.

INFORMATION MEDICINE HYPOTHESIS
Mode of transmission of therapeutic stimulus

Hypothesis that water and possibly other polar solvents can under certain conditions retain information about other substances with which they have previously been in contact, and which can be imparted to a sensitized biosystem.

OBSTACLE TO CURE
Factor preventing response to treatment

1. Factor in the nature of the disease process, or in the nature of the individual, or in his or her circumstances, habits or lifestyle that obstructs the response to well-indicated treatment.
2. Fixed or destructive state, external or internal to the individual, that prevents or undermines the healing process; including a psychological state.

ORGAN AFFINITY
Relationship of drug to organ

Some homeopathic medicines are particularly associated with specific organs whose disorders feature prominently in their materia medica. For example, Ceanothus is said to have an organ affinity with the spleen.

Comment. This concept is also applied in conventional medicine.

ORGANON
Organon of the rational art of healing

1. In its original Greek and Latin sense, an 'organ'; a morphic unit; any structural united collection of cells that is normally capable of coherently exercising a specific life-furthering function for the benefit of the greater whole – the individual body (Gaier H 1991 Thorsons' encyclopaedic dictionary of homeopathy. Thorsons, London).
2. Original statement of the principles of homeopathy, developed by Samuel Hahnemann through a series of six editions from 1810 to 1842.

ORTHODOX
Right thinking

Holding the right opinion.

Origin. Greek *orthos* = straight, correct, true; *doxa* = opinion.

Comment

1. Often used as synonymous with 'conventional', as in conventional medicine, but the two are not truly equivalent.
2. 'Orthodoxy' is so often claimed by separate elements of what is really a wider heterodoxy that it may be better to regard orthodoxy as a concept that represents a way of thinking based on discipline and integrity rather than a specific set of ideas.

PHARMACODYNAMICS
The pharmacological response at the receptor site

Determines the pharmacological response to the concentration of the drug at the active site. The presence and concentration of a drug at a site in the body is determined by its pharmacokinetics.

PHARMACOKINETICS
The behaviour of drugs in the body

The behaviour of a drug and its metabolites in the body over time.

PHENOMENOLOGY
Study of complete phenomena

1. The study, description and classification of phenomena.

2. The study of all the manifestations of an occurrence rather than of one circumscribed aspect of it or one particular view.
3. School of philosophy founded by Edmund Husserl, German philosopher 1859–1938.

Comment. Homeopathy adopts a phenomenological approach to illness. This is part of its holistic perspective. Both characteristics are opposed to the mechanistic or reductionist tendency inherent in the prevailing, conventional, pathophysiological medical model.

PLACEBO
Inert substance exerting therapeutic effect

1. A substance with no active biological properties knowingly or unknowingly used to exert a beneficial therapeutic effect. (Origin: Latin = 'I shall please'.)
2. An inactive agent used for comparison with the substance or method to be tested in a controlled trial.

PLURALIST HOMEOPATHY
Prescription of more than one drug

School or philosophy of homeopathic therapeutics using preparations of more than one homeopathic medicine in a single prescription representing different facets or levels of similarity. May describe the practitioner or the method.

Comment. Although the different medicines are prescribed together the instructions usually require that they are actually taken at different times, as distinct from complex or combination homeopathy, which uses fixed mixtures in a single dosage form.

Synonyms. Polypharmacy, polypragmasy.

POLYCHREST
Homeopathic drug of many uses

1. Commonly used homeopathic medicine with wide spectrum of therapeutic activity including all or nearly all systems of the body.
2. Homeopathic medicine of use in a wide range of morbidity.

Comment. The classification of a homeopathic medicine as a polychrest is to some extent dependent upon the scale of the

provings to which it has been submitted and the clinical
experience of its use, and hence the progress in the
development of its materia medica.

POTENCY
Active property of the drug

1. The biophysical property of a homeopathic medicine
   conferred by serial dilution with succussion, trituration or
   fluxion.
2. The degree of dilution achieved during the preparation of a
   homeopathic medicine, expressed as the number of serial
   dilutions and the proportionate dilution (decimal, centesimal,
   etc.) used in the series; thus 200C expresses the potency of the
   200th dilution of a centesimal series.

POTENTIZATION
Imparting therapeutic activity

1. The process by which the activity of a homeopathic medicine
   preparation is developed.
2. The process of serial dilution with succussion, including
   trituration or fluxion, employed in the production of
   homeopathic medicines from their 'stock'.

Comment. Potentization is not a defining characteristic of
homeopathic medicines. This is only and entirely based on the
similarity between the drug picture and the clinical picture; the
ability of the medicine to remedy a clinical condition similar to
that which it may induce in a healthy person.

PRIMARY DRUG ACTION
First phase of biological response to drug

1. The immediate impact of the medicine on the body.
2. Produces the expected effect of a material dose of the
   medicine. Thus it may increase (aggravate) the manifestation
   of the disorder in the patient.

PROFESSIONAL HOMEOPATH
Professionally qualified non-medical homeopath

Homeopathic practitioner who has undergone a prescribed
course of instruction (currently not formally defined or
regulated), but who is not a physician.

Comment. The legal status of these practitioners varies from country to country. In some EU states their practice is allowed, and indeed unregulated; in others it is illegal.

REPERTORY
Symptom–medicine cross-reference

Systematic cross-reference of symptoms and disorders to the homeopathic medicines in whose therapeutic repertoire they occur. The strength of the association between the two is indicated by the typeface in which the medicine name is printed.
Used in case analysis to identify the medicine indicated for the patient.

REPERTORIZATION
Use of repertory for decision support

The technique of using a repertory to identify the homeopathic medicines whose materia medica corresponds most closely to the clinical picture of the patient and from amongst which the similimum may be chosen.

Comment
1. Repertorization depends on accurate case analysis and the evaluation of symptoms that this involves so that the process is applied to those symptoms that are most significant in the individual patient.
2. Repertorization cannot be depended upon alone to identify the best prescription. It can only suggest possible choices. The prescriber's knowledge of the patient and the materia medica must determine the choice.
3. Computerized repertories are available that simplify the task of repertorization and allow more versatile analysis of the case.

RUBRIC
Key words identifying symptoms

The form of words identifying the symptom or disorder or its component elements and details within a repertory and to which a list of the relevant medicines is attached.

Comment. Repertorization requires that the patient's symptoms be expressed, 'translated' or interpreted in terms of the rubrics found in the repertory. This gives rise to the problem of 'repertory language' and its sometimes obscure relationship to the language of the patient.

SARCODE
Medicine derived from healthy tissue

Homeopathic medicine derived from healthy animal tissue or secretion, which has its own drug picture.

SECONDARY DRUG ACTION
Second phase of biological response to medicine

In this phase the reaction of the body to the medicine produces an effect contrary to the natural action of a material dose. Thus it relieves (remedies) the disorder in the patient.

SERIAL DILUTION
Sequence of dilutions

A sequence of separate and equal dilutions from the same stock, each accompanied by succussion or trituration.

SIMILE
Drug picture with likeness to clinical picture

Drug picture similar to the clinical picture.

Comment. There are different uses of the concepts of Simile and Similimum. The terms may be used synonymously, but the 'simile' concept is also used to describe a likeness between the drug picture and the clinical picture that is not as precise as the similimum and that may evoke a powerful response, possibly an aggravation, that does not lead to therapeutic change. On the other hand, the 'similimum' may be used to describe an exceptionally precise match, which evokes an exceptional response. The equivalence or difference between the two concepts remains a matter for debate.

SIMILIMUM
Drug picture most like clinical picture

1. The drug picture most like the clinical picture in the patient.

2. The most accurate match between clinical characteristics of the patient and the materia medica.
3. The basis of accurate and effective prescribing in homeopathy.

SINGLE DOSE
One dose of one medicine at one time

The principle of administering only one dose of a single medicine at any one time, further doses being dependent on the principles governing the repetition of the dose and the second prescription.

Comment. This is the basis of unicist homeopathy; often associated with the title of classical homeopathy.

SINGLE REMEDY
Single medicine prescription

Homeopathic prescription consisting of only one medicine derived from only one source material at one time.

SUCCUSSION
Shaking in between dilutions

1. Vigorous shaking, with impact or 'elastic collision', carried out at each stage of dilution in the preparation of a homeopathic potency.
2. Procedure of shaking the patient's body to elicit sounds of fluid in a body cavity or hollow organ.

TISSUE AFFINITY
Association of medicine with body tissue

The tendency for a homeopathic medicine to act on a particular type of body tissue. For example, Ruta has a special affinity for fibrous tissue.

TOXICITY, TOXICOLOGY
Poisonous properties of substances, study of toxic properties

The poisonous properties of substances, including drugs. The study of the poisonous effects of substances is the source of much homeopathic materia.

Comment. Many homeopathic medicines are derived from toxic substances. In low potency, where the medicine still contains a material dose of the toxic substance, the possibility of drug toxicity remains. Pharmaceutical regulations prohibit the sale of low potencies of homeopathic medicines derived from these sources.

Index